DOCTOR'S
CALL HOUR

DOCTOR'S CALL HOUR

by Beale H. Ong, M.D.

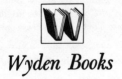

Wyden Books

First Edition

Trade distribution by Simon and Schuster
A Division of Gulf + Western Corporation
New York, New York 10020

Library of Congress Cataloging in Publication Data

Ong, Beale.
    Doctor's call hour.

    Includes index.
    1. Children—Care and hygiene—Miscellanea. 2. Children—Diseases—Miscellanea. I. Title.
RJ61.0528   618.9'2   77-17589
ISBN 0-671-22953-2

*In memory of my father, Harry A. Ong,
the finest physician I have ever known*

Contents

Acknowledgments

I would like to thank the following people for their contributions to this book. Without their unselfish help it would never have come into being.

My partners William A. Howard, M.D., Gordon W. Daisley, Jr., M.D., and Franklin L. Stroud, M.D., for their generosity in allowing me time away from the practice as well as for their many helpful suggestions.

For contributions in the areas of their specialties:

A. Barry Belman, M.D., Chief of Pediatric Urology, Children's Hospital National Medical Center (CHNMC)

Charles Broring, D.D.S., Chief of Pedodontics, CHNMC

Blackwell Brunner, M.D., Attending in Ophthalmology, CHNMC

Armand Dumas, D.D.S., Professor of Orthodontics, Georgetown University School of Dentistry

Gilbert Herer, Ph.D., Director, Children's Speech and Hearing Center, CHNMC

William A. Howard, M.D., Chief of Allergy and Immunology, CHNMC

Wellington Hung, M.D., Chief of Endocrinology, CHNMC

Stephen Nason, M.D., Associate Professor of Orthopedics, CHNMC

Peter Nigra, M.D., Chief of Dermatology, Washington Hospital Center

Robert A. Pumphrey, M.D., Attending in ENT, CHNMC

Judson Randolph, M.D., Chief of Pediatric Surgery, CHNMC

Lewis Scott, M.D., Chief of Pediatric Cardiology, CHNMC

For critical editorial review my special thanks to John L. Chamberlain, III, M.D., and Franklin L. Stroud, M.D.

To my loyal office staff, who pitched in whenever asked to type, duplicate, run to the post office, and put up with all the eccentricities of a neophyte author.

To Harry and Norma Stevens for their special help in making available a quiet and peaceful place in which to write during the long cold winter.

I am also deeply grateful to all those many parents who have participated in the call hour over the years and who continue to ring in each morning, not only because they have made this book possible, but more importantly because dealing with them and their offspring provides an ongoing experience for which I wouldn't trade places with anyone.

And most of all to my devoted wife Linn and our three children, Beale, Jr., John, and Carter, who gave me their whole-hearted support in this effort as they do in all others.

Dear Parents:

I recognize, of course, that there are many female pediatricians and other health-care specialists. I shall use "he," however, throughout in order to avoid the cumbersome repetition of "he or she." On the same principle I shall employ "he" to refer to all babies, even though half of them are female.

BEALE H. ONG, M.D.

DOCTOR'S
CALL HOUR

Introduction: "The Parents' Show and Tell Hour"

The questions on which this book is based are from my "call hour." Each morning from eight to nine o'clock I devote exclusively to answering any and all questions about children that I get from mothers and occasionally fathers. (I jot down those few which require some research before calling the parent back with what I hope will be a helpful answer.)

The scope of the questions truly reflects the broad and challenging specialty that pediatrics has become. It's potpourri; one mother calls it "the parents' show and tell hour"!

In checking with colleagues, I found that they too were the recipients of many of the same questions on a regular basis, and several recommended I pursue the task of collecting them—along with my answers. Still I was dubious about writing a book since I had neither desire nor time to add to the many that are published every year. But at the continued urging of patients' parents I finally decided to go further and see what had already been done in the way of books on child care. I read through one after another. I fully expected that a book such as this had already been done. To my surprise I found this not to be the case.

I found that many of the books were oriented along behavioral lines, written by psychologists, psychiatrists, and others who were not pediatricians. Still others were written from what I would call the academic point of view and lacked the practical aspects that are so necessary in day-to-day practice and direct patient responsibility. I felt quite firmly that there was a need for a new kind of book.

This is not to imply criticism of the work of others—much I felt to be of the highest quality—but many seemed to lose the reader in detailed dissertations about aspects of child rearing without offering very much in the way of practical advice. In other cases, advice was given which, after 12 years of practice, I found to be incorrect. Several others, while excellent at the time they were written, seemed out of date.

Finally, most were about what the author thought was important for parents to know, not about questions that parents really ask.

With the unselfish cooperation and wholehearted support of my partners in practice, I was able to free enough time to continue the task. My intention has been throughout the book to keep it brief and keep it practical. We have made so much of child rearing seem so complex and formidable as to appear downright impossible for parents. In the process, we have robbed ourselves of much of the enjoyment that goes with watching children develop instead of dissecting every move to see where on on some graph they will fall. The arts of trusting yourself and listening to what your conscience tells you have almost become lost!

The book has been organized into various sections with cross referencing and an exhaustive table of contents and index since I hope it will serve as a reference rather than as a volume which, once read, is discarded. It is with great humility that I present this work, for it is derived from my various teachers in pediatrics, including my late father, my partners in practice, my professors at the University of Pennsylvania and the Harvard Medical School's Boston Children's Hospital, as well as my colleagues at the Children's Hospital National Medical Center in Washington, D.C., all of whom have set the highest professional standards. So here it is: a book of questions that parents really do ask their pediatrician—and my attempts to answer them.

1

From Birth to First Birthday

CHECKING THE BABY AT BIRTH

What routine laboratory tests are done on the baby at birth?
The only routine test the baby receives is the PKU test. Other tests which are frequently (but not routinely) done are blood typing and bilirubin measurements.

What is PKU?
PKU is a rare metabolic disease (phenylketonuria) which, if left untreated, can cause mental retardation. All babies are tested in the hospital for this condition by means of a simple blood test. The incidence is somewhere around one in 15,000 births. It can be successfully treated by placing the infant on a special diet.

I have recently read where thyroid screening of newborn babies might be a good idea. What do you think?
Hypothyroidism, which can lead to mental deficiency, occurs in approximately one in 6000 births, and I think that we will soon be screening all babies for this condition. In fact, several newborn nurseries have already instituted this test on a routine basis.

What is the Apgar score that you hear so much about?
It is a means of rating the baby at one and five minutes after birth and includes heart rate, color, muscle tone, and respiratory effort. A rating from one to ten is used. Ten indicates the baby is

in perfect condition. Lower numbers serve to alert everyone that the baby has or may have difficulties.

I have recently heard of the so-called Brazelton scale. What is this?

This is a means of evaluating a baby's response pattern to various forms of stimulation and appears to aid early diagnosis of infants who may have later developmental difficulties. It was named for its originator, Dr. T. Berry Brazelton, a pediatrician and professor of pediatrics at the Harvard Medical School.

What kind of examination does the doctor do on a newborn baby?

Your doctor will do essentially the same type of examination that you would receive on your annual checkup. This includes examination of the head, eyes, ears, nose, and mouth, careful listening to the chest and heart sounds, feeling the abdomen, examination of the genitalia, the musculoskeletal system, and also a neurological examination. He will also check to see if the baby has urinated and make sure there is no rectal blockage. In addition to the physical examination he will carefully review the obstetrical record which records any complications in pregnancy, medications given, etc. He will also want to look carefully at the delivery room record to note anything which might affect the baby. He will note the Apgar score, and review any family history that might be pertinent, such as allergies, blood disorders, and the like.

HOSPITAL CARE

Are there any medicines which are routinely given to the baby while he is in the hospital?

Yes, two treatments are given to virtually all babies. The first is the placing of silver nitrate drops in the eyes to prevent gonorrheal infection which can cause blindness. The second is the injection of vitamin K to prevent infant death by sudden bleeding due to a deficiency of this vitamin.

What is a high-risk infant?

Babies born prematurely.

Babies born by Cesarean section or who have a difficult delivery.

Those born to mothers who have any sort of infection just prior to delivery or in some cases during pregnancy.

Infants born to mothers who are diabetic or who have other medical problems requiring close supervision.

Babies born to mothers who are in the older age group. Babies in these categories are frequently placed in a high-risk nursery or intensive-care nursery, if one is available. This is essentially a nursery area with a highly trained staff that can observe the baby closely for any signs of problems that may develop. Babies who appear ill at birth are, of course, also placed in this nursery.

I have heard that early contact between mother and baby is important. Is this true?

Yes, it certainly is. The maternal-child relationship begins immediately after birth and, therefore, even in the delivery room, holding and nursing of the baby, if possible, is desirable.

I understand that many important changes are taking place in newborn nurseries. Can you give me some idea what they are?

First of all, tremendous advances have been made recently in the care of so-called high-risk infants, which include sick babies as well as those who are premature or have other factors in their histories which make them more susceptible to difficulty. Various sophisticated monitoring devices, respirators, intravenous fluids, etc., have all made survival of these infants far more likely.

Secondly, we have become increasingly aware that the baby responds to his environment from the moment of birth. Nurseries are installing proper lighting, rocking and holding the babies, allowing parents free access to their infants whenever possible, encouraging talking to the baby, handling him, and the like. Gone, I hope, are the days when the baby was whisked away to the nursery and could only be seen during certain specified visiting hours.

My newborn baby seems to be so sleepy. He just doesn't seem interested in nursing, and yet my doctor has checked him and says that everything is OK.

Following the initial effort of being born into this world, which includes not only passage through the birth canal, but also the initial efforts of establishing and maintaining life on his own for the first time, he is plain tired out. For the first two or three days many babies sleep a great deal and many seem relatively uninterested in feeding, be it nursing or taking from a bottle. On approximately the third day, just as the breast milk begins to come in, they usually become more wakeful and from there on out activity picks up steadily. So don't worry, by the time you get him home he will be waking up frequently and hollering for the next feeding.

My baby has lost weight and he is only two days old. Is this cause for concern?

Not if he is otherwise acting well. All babies lose weight immediately following birth, up to 10 percent of the birth weight over the first few days.

How long should the baby stay in the hospital?

Barring complications I think that three days is a reasonable time. With a first baby I would prefer to have mother and baby stay at least this long since I think it makes for a smoother adjustment. I do feel that discharging the baby under 24 hours of age is not a good idea as many of the conditions such as jaundice and infection which cause us concern may not have had time to manifest themselves, nor can the PKU test be reliably done at such an early age.

How soon can I begin to nurse the baby?

Just as soon as you want to for all practical purposes—even in the delivery room.

What is a neonatologist?

He is a pediatrician who, upon completion of his general pediatric training, has taken additional formal training in diseases of the newborn. This program requires two years to complete and there is now a special board examination that certifies specialists in this area. More and more hospitals are adding neonatologists to their staffs, which has resulted in a great improvement in the care of the sick infant. When the baby is acutely ill the neonatologist often takes over, the pediatrician working right along with him.

What is a low-birth-weight baby?

Not long ago we used to say that any baby less than five and one-half pounds was a premature infant. Nowadays a distinction is made between the infant who is born before 36 weeks gestation and the full-term infant who is still small by weight. The first infant, the truly premature baby, is generally immature with respect to all body systems but has otherwise developed normally. The other infant, although mature, has suffered from retarded growth during the pregnancy. Approximately one-third to one-half of all small babies fall into this latter category. It is important to distinguish between these two types of infants since they are subject to different problems and therefore require different forms of care. For example, the low-birth-weight baby has a mature enough sucking reflex to do very well on the breast whereas the premature baby may have such an immature reflex as to make feeding via a nipple impossible.

How do you feel about circumcision?

Well over 90 percent of the male babies I care for are circumcised in the newborn period and I think it is generally a good idea. Certainly it makes local hygiene much easier and avoids the possible complications later on of adherence of the foreskin, which may necessitate circumcision at a later date. Certainly if you intend to have your son circumcised it should be done in the newborn period since it is accomplished quickly and easily and will be practically healed before he is discharged. If you wait until later it will necessitate a hospital admission, general anesthesia and, all in all, be a much more traumatic event. Don't worry about the lack of anesthesia for the infant; he won't remember it. Incidentally, I am often asked who performs the circumcision. The answer is the obstetrician, except of course in the case of a Jewish ritual circumcision, which is performed by a *mohel*. I might add that some of the best done circumcisions I have seen have been performed as part of the ritual service.

JAUNDICE

My baby was jaundiced in the hospital. What is jaundice?

Jaundice refers to a yellow color of the skin which is produced by elevated levels of bile pigment (called bilirubin) in the bloodstream. This is very common among newborn babies and usually causes no difficulty. Your doctor will order various blood tests to determine the cause of the jaundice—generally immaturity of liver function. Other types of jaundice are caused by blood group incompatibility, infection, or other more unusual metabolic disorders. Your doctor will keep track of the level of jaundice both by checking the infant periodically and by measuring bilirubin. In the majority of cases the jaundice clears within a few days without any specific treatment and causes no harm.

When can jaundice be dangerous in the newborn baby?

We are concerned when the bilirubin level, a laboratory measurement of the degree of jaundice, goes to high levels because, under rare circumstances, it may cause brain damage.

I have heard that some babies are put under a light when they are jaundiced. Is this true?

Yes, it certainly is. A few years ago when most nurseries had windows, the observation was made that those babies who were nearest the window and received more light were generally less jaundiced than others in the nursery. Studies documented this fact and it was decided to use artificial light to clear jaundice. A special light is used and the treatment is referred to as phototherapy. The baby is undressed and placed under the light for varying amounts of time, his eyes carefully covered to avoid any ocular damage. Phototherapy is very helpful in the management of many babies with jaundice in preventing the bilirubin from reaching potentially dangerous levels.

Is it true that exchange transfusions are now only rarely necessary?

Since the advent of Rhogam, an injectable antibody preparation, which is given to the Rh-negative mother and blocks the production of harmful antibodies, and the use of phototherapy, the need for exchange transfusion has been dramatically reduced.

Does the incidence of jaundice in newborn babies seem to be increasing?

Yes, it does. We assume that most cases of jaundice in the newborn are caused by so-called immaturity of liver function since this is the organ that normally clears the blood of bilirubin. There may well be some other as yet unknown factors involved, however, which are responsible for the apparent increase in this condition.

What about home deliveries?

There are just too many good reasons why having a baby in the hospital is so much better. Even in expected normal deliveries, emergencies can occur which require the use of special equipment, such as suctioning apparatus and oxygen. Why take an unnecessary chance with something so important?

TAKING HIM HOME

We are expecting our first child in about two months. Should we select a pediatrician in advance of his birth?

Yes, I think it is an excellent idea to select your pediatrician ahead of time. After all he is going to be a very important person to you both through the years. Many times your obstetrician will recommended a pediatrician. Occasionally the recommendation will come from friends whose judgment you trust or from the local hospital or medical society. Regardless of the source it is a good idea to call up and make an appointment for a prenatal visit to his office. More and more pediatricians are making themselves available for such get-acquainted conferences and I like the idea. During this initial meeting the prospective parents can ask various questions and have an opportunity to sense the general philosophy of the pediatrician.

I have just arrived home from the hospital with my new baby.
How should I follow through with the pediatrician?

He will have given you instructions during his visit to the
hospital along with a scheduled appointment for the baby at one
month of age. Checking in by phone during this period is a
great help in establishing good communication, which is the
touchstone of good medical practice. We ask our new mothers
to check in with us in the call hour two to three days after they
arrive home to give us a report. Thereafter we like to hear once
a week until the baby comes into the office for the first time.

Are there any danger signs to watch for when the baby gets home?

Yes, here are some with which you should be familiar:

Fever.

Sudden loss of appetite.

Poor color, especially any blueness—Many babies occasionally have a slight degree of blue color around the mouth
and occasionally of the hands and feet, but this is transient. If
blueness becomes more generalized, persists, or involves the
tongue, your doctor should see the baby.

Difficulty breathing, or choking while feeding.

Thick white coating of tongue or inside of mouth.

Vomiting—By this I mean actual vomiting and not
spitting up, which is something that many babies do in varying
amounts.

Muscular twitching—Most babies will startle with loud
noise or when moved quickly. This sort of tremor is of no consequence, but if they occur spontaneously while the baby is at
rest, this can be serious.

Diarrhea—Remember that breast-fed babies particularly
have loose, seedy, yellow, and frequent stools, eight to ten per
day, but if the stools become watery in consistency and are
passed with greater frequency and explosively this is a danger
sign.

Jaundice—if the baby becomes yellow in color or if the
jaundice noted in the hospital seems to be worsening, take the
baby in for a checkup.

Fever—A temperature of 100 degrees or under rectally is considered normal. Over this means a fever and you should call in. One note of caution here: occasionally small babies react to illness with a subnormal temperature (97 or below). This can also be a sign of illness and is actually more serious than a high temperature since it means that the body is not responding properly to the infection.

He doesn't look right—This is the most important sign of all. If there is some sudden change in the baby's behavior such as lethargy, poor feeding, or change of color, do not hesitate to check in with the doctor.

How do you feel about a baby nurse?

I think that the baby nurse often provides more interference than help. This is particularly true if you are nursing the baby and she has no role in feeding. Many times, because she feels left out, the nurse is not supportive of breast feeding. If you think you will need help with the new baby I'd suggest having someone come in to do the cleaning, cooking, etc., but who will leave the entire care of the baby up to you.

Is it all right to have pets around?

Yes, certainly, unless the baby happens to be born into a family where both parents have a strong history of allergy; then you may be asking for trouble. Long-haired dogs, as well as cats, are the worst offenders. Many mothers have asked me if there is a danger of a cat climbing into the baby's crib at night and smothering him. Although I have never read of this I think it a good general rule to keep pets out of the baby's room while he is sleeping or otherwise unattended.

How about visitors?

For the first two weeks restrict it to the family and for the first month adults are fine, but be careful of young children, who frequently have colds. I like to avoid taking the baby to crowded places such as supermarkets until he is at least two months old.

My parents want to come to see the baby as soon as I get home. They are planning to stay with us for a week or so. Is this a good idea?

Of course, it depends on your relationship with your parents, and your husband's as well. As a general rule, having grand-parents stay during the first two weeks or so is not such a good idea. In most cases, especially with the first baby, it takes some time for the new family unit to get off the ground. So, if you think there will be a tendency toward interference and tension, postpone the visit a bit.

What kind of mattress do you recommend for the baby's crib?

I generally prefer a firm mattress for all age groups. If it makes the parents' aching backs feel better, I suspect it does the same for the baby.

What about having a pillow in the crib or bassinet?

I wouldn't have one in the bed until the infant is at least six months old on the outside chance that it might fall over him and possibly suffocate him while sleeping.

When should he have his own room?

From the beginning. It is definitely not a good idea for the baby to sleep in your room if you can avoid it. He will adjust better in his own surroundings.

What temperature should I keep his room?

He might as well start right off adjusting to whatever temperature you like to maintain in your household and he'll do just fine.

When the new baby comes home can he sleep in my older child's room?

Unless the next oldest sibling is at least 3 to 5 years old the baby should preferably not sleep in the sibling's room. Small children, two to three years of age especially, may do bodily harm to the baby, either accidentally or even purposefully, so try not to leave the baby unattended with a child under three years of age. It's far better, whenever possible, to give the new baby his own room from the beginning. If this is not possible, have him sleep in your room.

When can he go outside?

He has already been outside on the way home from the hospital. So anytime thereafter is fine. Try to take him out every day. I'm a believer in the benefits of fresh, clean air, if you can find it.

BREAST-FEEDING

How do you feel about breast-feeding?

I am amazed at the number of parents who ask me this question. Some approach it as though what they are contemplating is illegal, dangerous, or even subversive. Keep in mind that the breasts are there primarily for this purpose.

I understand there has been an increase in the number of women who breast-feed. Do most of the mothers in your practice breast-feed their babies?

The overwhelming majority of mothers in my practice now breast-feed. I'm impressed not only with this increase but the higher success rate as well. The latter I attribute to the support new mothers receive from various parent groups and nursing personnel, particularly those in the newborn nursery. Lastly, the attitude of the pediatrician has been very important, as a knowledgeable and supportive physician greatly enhances the chances for successful breast-feeding.

Should I nurse the baby?

This is a very personal question and generalities are of no help in deciding which course of feeding to follow. My feeling is that in the long run there is little difference, if any, between the bottle- and breast-fed baby despite the myriad of studies done and the many articles written. I do believe, however, that the emotional satisfaction for both mother and baby is of paramount importance, and the mother must feel satisfied that she is doing the best thing for her infant no matter which method of feeding is chosen. I think that many mothers are made to feel that breast-feeding is too difficult and are therefore afraid to try. So much has been written extolling its virtues and spelling out in minute detail all sorts of helpful and at times unhelpful suggestions that this very natural process seems complex and difficult. Remember that the most primitive and uneducated peoples can do it, so why in the world can't you? Approach breast-feeding with a positive and relaxed attitude and the rest will take care of itself. Read extensively and worry constantly and you haven't got a chance. But, if nursing doesn't work out, keep in mind that it was nursing that was a failure, not you.

Are there any tips on increasing the breast milk supply?
    Yes, the following suggestions should be helpful:
        Drink plenty of fluids (at least three quarts per day), and remember it can be any kind of fluid; milk doesn't make milk, and beer has no special effect.
        Make sure you are taking in about 1000 calories over your usual diet.
        Most important of all, get plenty of rest and relax and enjoy! The amount of milk is inversely proportional to the amount of worry!

Can I nurse my premature infant?
    Frequently you will be able to nurse him unless he is so small that he will not suck well enough or unless he is ill. Most nurseries are very cooperative and will allow mothers to come in and feed their babies at any time, an enlightened attitude that has been a long time coming.

My premature infant is too small to nurse from the breast. Is it possible to give him breast milk that I express with a pump?
    Pediatricians and more particularly neonatologists are more and more coming around to the view that even very small premature infants may do well on breast milk if it is "spiked" with a few extra ingredients.
How long will breast milk keep?
    When stored promptly in the refrigerator it can be kept up to 72 hours. The milk may also be frozen and kept for an inde-

finite period. I don't advise doing this, however, as I fear some degradation in quality during the freezing process.

What are some reasons for failure of breast-feeding?

First and foremost, too much anxiety about the whole thing!

Not enough rest.

Insufficient fluid and/or caloric intake.

Lack of an informed and/or supportive nurse, physician, friend, or grandparent.

An occasional infant who will not take to the breast.

What medications should I avoid while nursing?

Almost all medication will appear in the breast milk; it is therefore a wise policy to check with your pediatrician if you are taking, or plan to take, any form of medication.

Can I return to work and continue to nurse the baby?

You bet! If you're close enough to come home for a feeding you've got it made. If not, you can try using a breast pump while you're at the office if you are uncomfortable. The longer you have been nursing, the longer the possible interval between feedings. Some mothers can nurse three or four times a day quite successfully after they have been nursing for three to four months.

How long should I nurse him?

As long as you and he are enjoying it. In my practice the average is four to six months. By then most antibody transfer has taken place and nutritionally he will do well on bottle or breast, so that the deciding factor should be how long you feel comfortable.

I would like to nurse but my breasts are small.

You will be pleasantly surprised to hear that the size of the breast has no bearing on the amount of milk you can produce.

Can I nurse my twins?

Yes, you certainly can, and both at the same time, too!

Is a nipple shield all right to use?

Yes, you want to avoid getting too sore at first; later on you can discontinue it.

How frequently should I nurse him?

An excellent question. I advise nursing about every three hours for the first week or two and then dropping back to a four-hour interval. The exception to this is that if the baby sleeps from midnight to 6 A.M., for goodness sake, don't wake him as your rest is more important in enhancing the milk supply. Nursing more frequently than every three hours usually produces soreness of the nipples (which can be helped by a topical application of vitamin E), which will then inhibit milk production and does not give sufficient time for the breast to refill. Also, the infant will not be sufficiently hungry after a short interval to do the vigorous sucking necessary to stimulate the milk supply. A very frequent mistake is to let the baby sleep for long periods in the daytime. This usually means that he is not getting enough and has given up trying. Don't fall into this trap of infrequent nursing, which further diminishes the milk supply and quickly results in the formation of a vicious cycle. It is better to wake him and nurse him at regular intervals, which will serve to stimulate milk production.

How will I know if he is getting enough?

First of all, if he seems content and wakes regularly for his feedings he's probably doing fine. You will probably experience a feeling of engorgement, especially prior to the feeding. If he is constantly chewing on his fist, continues to want to suck vigorously after finishing at the breast, or continues to fuss he is probably not getting enough. Also, watch out for the baby who, especially in the first few weeks, nurses five to ten minutes and then falls asleep. Frequently he is not getting enough, but instead of loudly protesting, having found on several previous occasions that nothing more was forthcoming, he'd just as soon quit and go back to sleep. This kind of guy may then sleep six or seven hours at a stretch. If you have any doubt about the situation the sensible thing to do is to offer some sugar water immediately after nursing him. If he gobbles down five or six ounces at a crack, then he's hungry. If he doesn't take any and you are still doubtful, try some formula after one or two nursings since an occasional baby will not take water. And don't worry about an occasional bottle disrupting nursing. On the contrary, it might save the day!

When can I give a relief bottle?

It's best to wait until the nursing is well established, which usually takes about two weeks. You can then add a bottle in place of the 2 A.M. feeding, which will also give his father a chance at trying his skill. Adding formula too soon and too frequently will quickly lead to a diminished milk supply.

How long do I have to nurse my baby in order to ensure that he has gotten all the antibodies from my milk?

Colostrum, the premilk secretion from the breast, is rich in antibodies and after the first few weeks of nursing the amount of antibody transmitted decreases. We still do not know how long the process of antibody transfer continues nor exactly what different types are concentrated in breast milk. Generally speaking this process continues for a longer period of time and is far more complex in terms of the different types of antibodies transmitted than previously thought.

I have read a lot recently regarding the dangers of polychlorinated biphenyls (PCB) in breast milk and their potentially harmful effects on the baby. Is it safe to continue breast-feeding?

Yes, the consensus is that it is prefectly reasonable and in fact highly desirable to continue breast-feeding. Although we are concerned about the presence of PCBs in the environment, there is not enough justification to discontinue what we know to be such a valuable thing for the mother and the baby.

I have heard that if my infant is breast-fed his skin will be more sensitive and he will develop more rashes. Is this true?

No. In fact, the chances of allergic rashes are lessened by breast-feeding.

I am going to have a Cesarean section. Will I be able to nurse my baby?

Yes, there is no reason why you won't be successful, so plan on it!

What else helps milk production?

Rest, rest, and more rest. It is by far the most important factor in successful breast-feeding. This means emotional as well as physical relaxation. Regular naps are often helpful in the early stages, as is a reasonably predictable schedule of feeding.

May an infant be allergic to breast milk?

This occasionally happens. Such an allergy may produce a rash or colic.

What are some reasons for diminished milk supply?

Not enough rest.

Nursing too long or too frequently.

Insufficient fluid intake.

Insufficient relaxation—too much worry about "will I be successful?"

Not enough caloric intake.

Letting the baby sleep for prolonged periods of time and therefore giving the breast insufficient stimulation to produce milk.

Misinformation and/or lack of support from family, friends, and even health-care professionals.

Giving too many supplemental bottles before the breast milk supply is securely established.

I am nursing my baby and everything was going along just fine until he got two teeth and now he occasionally bites. What can I do?

The obvious answer is, of course, to wean him from the breast, and, assuming he is five or six months old, this may be an excellent idea.

If you very much want to continue nursing try the following. When he clamps down too hard, withdraw the nipple from his mouth immediately and let out a loud "ouch." Tell him that it hurt. Many times he will quickly get the idea that biting produces an unpleasant interruption in his feeding and will stop the nasty habit. Babies are a whole lot smarter than we give them credit for being!

May I diet while breast-feeding?

Dieting will not have a bad effect on the milk supply if the mother is overweight and continues to follow the other rules for good milk production.

I have just come down with a nasty cold. Is it all right to continue to nurse the baby?

In most instances it is perfectly all right to go ahead. After all, since the baby is going to get exposed no matter how you feed him and since colds (upper respiratory infections) are spread through the air it makes no difference. You should check with your pediatrician regarding other types of infections and be particularly careful not to take certain medications which might be transmitted through the breast milk and possibly be harmful to the baby. If you are running a fever and feel really knocked out for the first day or so, it is best to use formula for 24 or 48 hours. The breast supply often drops off during this period, but usually there is no difficulty in resuming after a short time.

I am nursing my baby and the doctor has said I will need a chest X-ray because I may have pneumonia. Is there any chance that radiation will be subsequently transmitted to my baby via the breast milk?

No. The small amount of radiation you receive during the chest film is quickly dissipated and there is no chance any will be transmitted to the infant.

How long should he nurse at each feeding?

For the first two to three days you should keep the nursing time to five to ten minutes on each side. Remember that the milk usually doesn't come in until the third day and that you want to avoid getting too sore before it does. Gradually over the next one to two weeks build up to 20 to 30 minutes on one side and five to ten on the other, alternating breasts at each feeding. You will find that each feeding will take approximately 45 minutes. Prolonged nursing, over an hour, is not necessary. The baby gets 90 percent of the milk in the first five to ten minutes and the remainder of the time is spent in meeting his sucking needs. It's interesting that after nursing is well established the time of feeding gradually decreases and many mothers find that they can successfully nurse their four- or five-month-old infant in less than ten minutes. Just remember to build up gradually and to alternate sides.

What foods should I avoid when breast-feeding?

Chocolate, nuts, and shellfish are best avoided. Heavy green vegetables such as kale and brussels sprouts can also produce considerable gassiness in the baby and highly spiced foods are, of course, not a good idea, so save that Indian curry recipe and avoid the Mexican restaurants for a while. Recently there has been considerable interest in cow's milk allergy as a cause of gassiness in the nursing baby. I have tried with some success to eliminate milk and milk products from the maternal diet in situations where the baby continued to be "colicky" despite the deletion of the common offenders noted above. Whenever a breast-fed baby is gassy or colicky one should first suspect something in the maternal diet. A cocktail and/or a glass of wine is certainly permissible; whatever amount comes through in the breast milk will probably soothe his nerves as well as yours. Contrary to folklore, however, drinking beer does not increase the milk supply. It never ceases to amaze me me how rapidly what you eat can be transmitted to the infant via the breast milk. I am convinced that the effects may be noted within two to four hours and last from 24 to 48 hours.

Instead of using a formula for the supplemental bottle I wonder if it would be all right to express some breast milk manually and keep it on hand for those occasions?

It certainly is permissible. Just put it in a thoroughly cleaned bottle and you may store it in the refrigerator for 48 to 72 hours.

What is so-called breast-feeding jaundice?

This type usually begins at the end of the first week or two and is usually quite mild and of no consequence. It is almost never a reason to discontinue breast-feeding, although occasionally your doctor may want the baby off the breast for a short period and may want him to take additional fluid in the form of sugar water to help "wash out" the bilirubin.This is particularly likely when the breast-feeding jaundice is superimposed on one of the other types. Occasionally he may even want to determine a bilirubin level to judge the degree of jaundice. This is a simple blood test which can be performed in many doctors' offices or at a nearby laboratory. The result should be available in an hour or two.

I am nursing the baby, but plan to have the sitter give him a bottle when we are out. How much should I give him?

As much as he wants, up to a full eight ounces.

How should I go about weaning him?

Gradually, so as to avoid discomfort on your part as well as his. Replacing one nursing with a bottle every three to four days usually works beautifully. Begin with the last feeding of the day and work backward since it is the early morning feeding when he is the hungriest and your milk supply is the greatest. Usually there is no need for any medication to help "dry up the milk" if weaning is done gradually. And don't worry if he doesn't take right to the bottle. When he gets hungry enough he will.

BOTTLE-FEEDING

How much should I feed him?

This of course varies with both the size and age of the baby. As a general rule he will tell you when he is getting full by fidgeting, arching backward, pushing the bottle away, and generally acting bored.

Some guidelines which may be helpful include the following:

By the time he gets home from the hospital he may be

taking as much as four ounces of formula at a crack. If he hollers for more, go ahead and give it to him.

Don't invest in four-ounce bottles that he will outgrow as fast as he later will shoes. Start with the eight-ounce variety.

At three to four months of age, when solids may be first introduced, he will take up to one-half a baby food jar of each food offered and by four to six months of age three-quarters to a full jar of fruit, vegetables, meat, etc., per feeding, depending on the variety offered to him.

Is a schedule advisable and if so what kind?

Yes. One that is predictable and fits into your household routine is best. In talking about schedules, the basic point to keep in mind is that *all* babies tend to wake up early for their feedings. They know a good deal early in life and are quick to take advantage of it. The nutritional satisfaction is only one part; babies enjoy being held and talked to, and why not? The more of this they can get the better as far as they are concerned. So what they do is wake up early and act starved! All right so far, but what then? They will often nurse only a few minutes or take only an ounce of formula and then go back to sleep, only to wake up an hour later, screaming. For the breast-fed baby this does not often give enough time for the breast to refill because the more frequent the feeding the less the supply, and of course maternal soreness may also lead to difficulty. Whether the baby is being breast-fed or formula-fed this frequent feeding at unpredictable intervals can lead to considerable maternal (and paternal) fatigue.

To prevent the cycle from getting started I usually advise that the baby not be fed more frequently than every three hours. Be arbitrary for a few days in the beginning and you will have an easy time thereafter. Let him outsmart you and it will be doubly hard to develop a schedule later on. If he wakes early for a feeding try letting him fuss for a few minutes and see if he won't settle down. If this fails, then often a diaper change may be helpful. If he persists, then I recommend offering some tap water with a bit of sugar added (one-quarter teaspoon to four ounces water). The sugar is necessary since most babies will have nothing to do with plain water. These attempts to "hold him off" for a time will ensure that he will have a good appetite at the next feeding. He will then take more from the breast or bottle and be more content immediately following the feeding and then sleep for a longer interval before the next. In summary my feeling is that a middle ground between a rigid arbitrary schedule and complete unpredictability is best. It is often very important to keep the family's overall schedule in mind. The routine and uniform principles of scheduled feedings no longer apply in today's family, where both parents are so much on the go. Each family must develop its own pattern of regularity.

I have recently heard that there is a move away from feeding infants cow's milk. Could you tell me something about this?

Many nutritionists and pediatricians feel that cow's milk may not provide the infant with optimum nutrition for the following reasons:

1. It does not provide the infant with the optimum ratio of protein and fat.

2. Vegetable oil is the source of fat in most commercial infant formulas and this has been shown by various investigators to be more efficiently absorbed by babies than the butterfat in cow's milk. The fat in human milk is the most easily absorbed of all.

3. Cow's milk is naturally deficient in iron.

4. Cow's milk allergy is very common and recent studies have shown that it may cause an allergic reaction in the lining of the intestine which results in microscopic amounts of bleeding (not visible to the naked eye). This chronic blood loss may cause depletion of the baby's iron stores.

5. The incidence of symptoms such as gassiness, spitting up, and genral fussiness due to cow's milk intolerance is quite high and is the cause of "colic" in numerous babies.

If the baby is allergic to whole milk, might he be able to tolerate skimmed milk?

No, if he is allergic to cow's milk in one form he will react to it in any other form. Besides, we do not think that giving skimmed milk to babies is a good idea. (See page 27.)

Should I warm the milk before giving it to the baby?

I favor warming the milk since it seems more natural, at least in the first few months. Breast milk arrives already warmed to body temperature.

If I mix different types of bottles, for example, the standard glass bottles and those with disposable inserts, will this give the baby any problem?

No, it should not.

Do you prefer the old-fashioned type of bottle or the newer type with the disposable insert?

I don't think it makes the least bit of difference which type you use. In my experience the disposable type doesn't help the "gassy" baby any more than the conventional bottle. Just make sure you get eight-ounce bottles, as he will graduate to this amount before you can bat an eyelash.

What about sterilization? Is it necessary?

I no longer advise routine sterilization but do caution that the bottles be washed carefully (along with the nipples) in hot water, preferably in the dishwasher. In hot weather one must be particularly careful not to let the bottle sit out because bacteria can grow much faster in the formula at warmer temperatures. In areas where overall sanitation may be a problem, such as where well water is used, sterilization in the first few months of life is certainly a good idea.

Is it all right to prop up the baby's bottle when I feed him?

No, this is a bad idea although convenient at times. The baby gets a great deal of emotional input during the feeding time from the closeness of being held and talked to; don't deprive him of any of it.

What are bottle caries?

These are caries (cavities) produced by excessive use of the bottle, particularly at nap and bedtime, in which case milk or juice is allowed to pool around the teeth, particularly the front teeth, which leads to early tooth decay. Putting the child to bed with a bottle is therefore to be avoided.

Is it necessary for him to burp after every feeding?

No, it is not. Some babies burp frequently and easily, others little or not at all. If he is content and happy, don't be concerned.

What about skimmed milk? You hear so many bad things about fat in whole milk. I don't want a weight problem.

Most babies belong on whole milk, but you are quite right about not wanting a fat baby. It wasn't so long ago that a fat baby was supposed to be nice and healthy but we know better now. Fat babies are no better off than fat adults. Frequently a reduction or delay in the addition of solid food that may be pushed at him in too great a quantity at too early an age is all that is needed. Skimmed milk will not meet the growth requirements of the baby under one year of age because it is simply too low in calories. It is also deficient in iron and essential fatty acids and for these reasons we do not recommend that skimmed or so-called fortified skimmed milk be used during the first year of life.

In my practice overfeeding is far more of a problem and all of us must resist the temptation to stuff the baby! This business of equating successful mothering with how much food can be gotten into him has got to go. Remember, most of today's grandparents were raised at a time when we were not aware of what good nutrition was and therefore may have ideas to the contrary. Roll with the punches but stick to your guns; more and more we are learning that we are a product of what we eat.

When should he be off the bottle?

Most babies are pretty well off the bottle by 18 to 20 months of age. The following is a good schedule. Start juice from the cup at six to eight months of age. Then, replace the midday bottle with a cup at 8 to 12 months. The next bottle to go is the evening one and this is best done somewhere around 14 to 16 months. The morning bottle stays the longest because that is when he is really hungry and therefore enjoys it most. There are variations of course, but the main thing to remember is that there is a normal developmental thrust away from sucking as a means of nourishment. Prolonged use of the bottle after the age of two years is not a good idea since it has ceased to be a means of nourishment and has become associated only with emotional satisfaction. Usually most infants are happily off the bottle at 20 to 24 months of age. If the baby breast-feeds as long as six months or more, it is often not necessary to wean to a bottle, and then have to go through another weaning process later. Usually, around 6 to 8 months, babies are quite eager to drink from a cup (and adept at it), at least at mealtimes.

OTHER FOODS

Can you give me some idea as to what foods to start when?

The most recent trend in infant feeding is to delay the intro-duction of solid food until four to six months of age. Occasionally, however, a younger baby will take such a large volume of milk that he is uncomfortable and solid food such as cereal enables him to obtain some concentrated calories that don't add lots of volume to his tummy. For most babies I like to start solids as follows:

Cereal—A good source of iron, rice is the least likely to cause trouble and can be started twice a day, in the morning around eight or nine and in the evening around 6 P.M. Mix with a little breast milk or formula to make it the consistency of paste and use the baby spoon rather than adding it to the bottle. For the most part I start this about four to six months of age.

Fruit—This is usually begun a month later. Peaches, pears, apricots, and prunes tend to be laxative foods but are not as allergenic as bananas and apples, which also tend to be more constipating. Give twice a day along with the cereal but not mixed together.

Vegetables—Yellow vegetables are less likely to cause trouble and are therefore begun first: squash, carrots, sweet potato, corn, and cauliflower. After two to three weeks green vegetables may be introduced. These are given in the middle of the day and are started one month after the introduction of fruit.

Meat—Start one month after vegetables. Lamb and veal produce the fewest difficulties. Give in the middle of the day with vegetables.

Egg yolk—This is usually begun one month later. The egg yolk may either be fresh or jarred. It should be given in the morning with cereal and fruit. Recently there has been great concern regarding egg yolks and cholesterol. Unless you have a positive family history of abnormally high cholesterol levels there is no harm in giving egg yolk to the baby. More about this when we discuss it later.

Juice—I like to begin juice by offering it in the afternoon around 3 P.M. Rotate apple, pineapple, and orange juice and don't forget many times he may settle for plain water. You may use "adult" juice from the beginning. One word of caution here. Babies often love juice, particularly apple, and these apple juice addicts, will drink unlimited amounts of the stuff! Mothers then wonder why they won't take any other foods offered. The amount of natural sugar even in unsweetened apple juice can cause rampant dental caries. So beware and use in moderation! It is not necessary that the baby have juice every day, and never offer more than a total of six ounces.

Desserts—It would probably be a fine idea never to introduce them at all, but if you do, try to stay away from the high-carbohydrate ones. He will learn about ice cream, cake, doughnuts, etc., soon enough!

In summary my policy is to add cereal, fruit, vegetables, meat, egg yolk, and juice all at one-month intervals. With the addition of egg yolk I like to give meat twice a day and cereal only in the morning. If you were to rank the foods in order of the baby's preference it would come about as follows: fruit, cereal, yellow vegetables, green vegetables, egg yolk, and meat.

It is a good idea to wait three to four days after the introduction of each individual food for the first time to make sure that it fully agrees with him and isn't going to produce diarrhea, excessive gassiness, vomiting, or a rash. By following this approach you can save yourself a lot of grief by immediately being able to pinpoint the offending food. Otherwise, you may have to resort to an elimination technique in order to find the culprit.

When should I introduce table food?

Usually about eight months of age. Begin by placing small pieces of food (things he can't choke on) such as banana, soft cheese, and the like on the feeding table and let him take it from there. Often it is better to feed him a bit yourself initially to get rid of those hunger pangs and then in the middle of the mealtime present him with some table food. If he doesn't want anything to do with it, back off for a couple of weeks before trying again. There is no reason to rush him.

How do you feel about fresh versus prepared baby foods?

I prefer fresh food, but I also realize that at times convenience will take precedence.

Have there been any recent changes in baby foods to bring them into line with current nutritional research? For example, what about added salt and sugar?

Yes, the major manufacturers of baby foods have made several recent and significant changes to improve their products. They have eliminated or are in the process of eliminating added salt from their foods. Remember that the baby does need some salt and most foods contain some naturally but it is the added salt that is considered potentially harmful, possibly contributing to high blood pressure later in life.

The amount of sugar in baby foods has also been curtailed and will only be added to those which, sugarless, are too unpleasant to the taste buds; for example, peaches and apricots.

Generally, the baby foods manufactured by the three major companies contain no artificial flavorings or colors, preservatives, or flavor enhancers.

Continue to read the labels carefully, but recognize that the area of nutrition is undergoing rapid changes and there will be new developments almost daily.

Is it necessary to heat solid foods?

I think most of them are more palatable to babies if they are warmed.

How long can I keep baby food after it has been opened?

It will keep in the refrigerator up to 72 hours. The same is true with formula, providing it has not been allowed to stand out at room temperature for more than an hour.

Why has the baby stopped taking milk?

This is often the case at six to eight months of age. By this time he frequently shows a considerable interest in solid foods, which will gradually begin to take precedence over milk.

How early can he have teething biscuits?

I would rather not give them to him at all. He really doesn't need those calories between meals, and I am convinced that this begins the snack habit that can have such disastrous consequences later on. He will be just as content teething on one of the many objects designed for this purpose. These can be reused and won't add calories at the wrong times.

My child was placed on a milk-free diet because he appears to be allergic to it. What about calcium? I am afraid he will not get a sufficient amount?

Good question. Your doctor may need to prescribe supplemental calcium if he feels it is indicated. Some good dietary sources include collards, turnip greens, spinach, broccoli, blackstrap molasses, kale, soybeans, and rhubarb. Frequently such children may be able to tolerate some dairy products in the diet, such as cheese and yogurt.

What are some foods that contain iron?

Fortified cereal, cooked beef, chicken, lamb, ham, liver, dried peaches, dried prunes, prune juice, eggs, raisins, spinach, tuna fish, scallops, shrimp, veal, watermelon, wheat germ, strawberries, cooked turkey.

Is it true that I should avoid adding extra salt or sugar to the baby's foods?

Yes, it is true. We are concerned that too much salt may predispose the infant to the development of hypertension (high

blood pressure) later on, and of course excess sugar will add un-
wanted calories as well as contribute to dental caries. It looks as
though the natural sugar and salt in basic foods is sufficient, and
although occasional additions are permissible, excessive use is to
be discouraged.

Are vitamins necessary?

Yes, they are. Supplemental vitamins are needed for the
breast-fed infant. Most of the time the diet for other children is
sufficient to provide needed vitamins, except for those infants who
take cow's milk and not enough other fortified foods. For the child
over two who is eating a balanced diet supplemental vitamins are
not needed. Most children in this country can discontinue them
even earlier. This is, however, an individual matter and depends
on each child's diet.

Does my baby need iron?

Yes, he does. Recently, iron-fortified formulas have come into
widespread use, but they frequently seem to cause stomach upset
and colicky behavior and therefore I do not prescribe them on a
routine basis. For the breast-fed as well as formula- or milk-fed
baby it is important to introduce some iron-containing solids.
Cereal is the best at about four months of age. Meat and egg yolk
are also good sources of iron. It is about this time when the iron
stores present at birth are about used up. All babies should have
a hemoglobin determination done some time in the first year,
usually around eight months, to make sure that they have sufficient iron stores.

What about cholesterol in the diet?

There are a few instances when elevation of blood cholesterol
and other fats may be hereditary. Unless the infant has been
documented as having one of these conditions, no restriction is
necessary.

Can a baby be overweight?

You bet he can. Recent studies have shown that the number
of fat cells is partially determined in the first few months of life.

The more fat cells, the more the tendency to be overweight for the rest of one's life. A fat baby is no healthier than a fat adult.

If this is true should I try to keep him on the underweight side?

No. Recent investigations have shown that nutritional deprivation and lack of proper weight gain and linear growth may be associated with decreased brain development. One must therefore walk a careful line between the two extremes.

SLEEPING

Can you suggest reasonable bedtime hours for different ages?

Here's a general schedule that I think will be helpful:

—2 months—By six to eight weeks of age he should be sleeping through from 10 or 11 P.M. until 6 A.M. No 2 A.M. feeding!

3–5 months—By four to five months of age he should be sleeping from 7 P.M. until 6 or 7 A.M. He may need some encouragement to drop that 10 P.M. bottle but don't be afraid to give him a little.

—2 years—To age two 7 to 7:30 is a reasonable hour for bedtime.

3–5 years—For the preschooler 8 P.M. seems about right.

6–9 years—8:30 to 9.

10–12 years—9:30.

13–Up to 10:30, occasionally later, depending on the homework, etc., but not every night.

Take all this with a grain of salt. It is not meant to be binding but it does give you some idea as to when junior should retire.

When should he sleep through the night?

Usually never, unless he gets a little help! On the average a baby should sleep from 10:30 to 6:00 A.M. at about four to six weeks of age. The only way to find out if he will is to gamble and not go in for the 2 A.M. feeding if he doesn't wake up. If he then awakens at 3 or 4 A.M. you can try to change his diaper and put him down again; he will often go back to sleep. If he persists in crying try a little water and if this doesn't do the job you've temporarily lost the battle. Wait another three to four days and try again. If after six to eight weeks he is not sleeping through the night (which means that you aren't either), then you must take the cold turkey approach and prepare yourself for what usually turns out to be three to four nights of yelling before the *habit*, for that is what it is by now, is broken. Keep in mind that there is just no good reason why a healthy full-term baby needs to eat at such an hour and that not feeding him in the middle of the night isn't going to do any harm to his psyche. Quite the contrary, overfatigued parents whose nerves are frayed are far harder on his emotional well-being.

How long should the baby stay awake?

Waking time gradually increases with age. During the first three to four weeks most babies are back to sleep just about as soon as the completion of the feeding. By six weeks they are awake for 30 minutes to an hour afterward. The more the higher centers of brain function develop, the more the infant obtains from his environment and the longer the waking period becomes.

He rolls over at night and then cries. Now what?

This little maneuver is analogous to the cat up the tree. Fortunately, he will soon learn to roll back again, but until he does you're stuck, and will just have to go ahead and perform this task for him.

What if he won't go to sleep at nap time?

Most babies will nap twice a day from four to six months of age to one year and once a day, usually in the afternoon, after the first birthday and continuing up to the age of three to four years. The amount of time will vary as will the degree of sleep, from none at all to being thoroughly "zonked." If the baby and the rest of the family are happy with the sleep schedule, then, whatever the pattern is, within reason, so be it.

I do believe that all infants, as well as older children, need a certain amount of time to themselves in order to recuperate and also to develop their own creativity. To my way of thinking the term *nap* should describe a distinct period during the day when the infant or toddler is to be left alone, preferably in his bed or at least in his own room. What he does during this time, within reason, is his business. One must also not forget the beneficial effect this period has on whichever parent might be at home that day. A little R and R for mother or father is just as necessary as it is for baby and these times of separation are necessary, positive experiences for both.

I find that failure to achieve proper sleep cycles is generally due to too high a level of stimulation. Too much TV and too many toys, mobiles, weekend trips, play groups, etc. An infant, like an adult, if overstimulated becomes chronically fatigued, which leads to more irregular sleep patterns and to poorer quality sleep, all of which continues the vicious cycle. Overextension of the nap period can also cause difficulties. Where both parents work, some helpers in the home or day care facilities may find that prolonged or frequent napping is the easy way out. This can result in understimulation of the infant and therefore hamper his development.

The baby was sleeping beautifully at night but now is waking up and crying for no apparent reason. Why?

This frequently occurs somewhere from five to eighteen months of age. Believe it or not it is due to dreaming, a phenomenon which few people realize begins in infancy. It is best to go in the room and satisfy yourself that he's OK. Give him a pat and get out quickly. Don't offer him something to eat. He'll act starved, but that is *not* the reason he has awakened. Feeding him, a frequent mistake, will only serve to condition him to expect a nice snack in the middle of the night.

He sleeps beautifully in the daytime but he is awake all night.

All babies like to turn night into day. It seems as though they always stay just one step ahead of you! The best way to handle this is to try to awaken him for a feeding about every three to four hours during the day. If he shows no interest, don't give in at night. Let him fuss, try a change of diapers, and perhaps a little sugar water. Stay with it for two to three nights and you will soon have things turned right way around.

It may sound silly, but I am a great believer in talking to babies in a fairly sophisticated manner. When he wakes in the middle of the night just tell him that this just isn't necessary and you are going to call a halt to it. Perhaps it's the tone of voice, but this speechmaking frequently works!

I have noticed that the baby's breathing is occasionally jerky, particularly when he is sleeping. Is this all right?
In the first few weeks of life the baby's breathing is often irregular at times. If his color is good, he feeds well, and in all other respects seems normal it is most often nothing to be concerned about.

Should my baby sleep on his back or stomach?
Babies prefer to sleep on their stomachs and seem to sleep more soundly this way. This is also a safer position should the infant unexpectedly vomit during sleep since he is less likely to inhale the vomitus in this position.

Should he sleep in the infant seat?
No. He will prefer his bed, which is more familiar to him. Furthermore, sleeping for prolonged periods of time with his feet curled up and propped up in a seat puts weight on the legs and may tend to accentuate the normal bowing of the legs at this age.

GENERAL BEHAVIOR

How do you distinguish between normal crying and crying that can mean something more serious?
Usually picking him up and cuddling him will give you the answer. Frequently that's all he wants and he will settle down promptly. Babies can be "spoiled" in this regard as early as a few weeks of age. They catch on to a good thing fast! If picking him up doesn't do the trick try changing his pants; if this is not successful he may be hungry and you should try giving him some milk. If he persists in crying he may well have a problem that needs medical attention and you should check in with your pediatrician.

Can my baby sleep too long?

Ordinarily, if the baby otherwise seems happy and content and is growing, the answer is no. There are two situations where a baby's prolonged periods of sleep deserve to be mentioned. The first is that rare instance where the baby may not receive sufficient environmental stimulation. The second is the occasional baby who's being breast-fed and who sleeps for very long periods of time between feedings because he is *not* getting enough breast milk.

Should I let him cry?

If there is nothing that you can determine that's wrong with him and he stops immediately when you pick him up, then it's his way of asking for more attention. When you feel that you've had enough and do not want to play with him, do what your conscience dictates and let him fuss. He's got to learn sooner or later that all his demands are not going to be met when he wants them and occasionally not at all. So why not begin to teach him from the beginning? It's far easier for a baby to learn to handle frustration at an early age than suddenly to be required to handle it later on—he's not going to get rid of that teacher he doesn't like and he'll have to take that required math course.

He always seems to fuss in the evening.

He sounds like a normal baby. From 5 to 9 P.M is the peak crying time. I call it the "sour hour." It is the end of the day, with the highest noise levels, siblings in the kitchen, TV, maternal fatigue, dinner to cook, and father home, hungry, and wanting to read the paper. The baby joins right in to add his contribution to the chaos that reigns in most homes at this time. What to do? Grin and bear it, for it's a passing stage. Don't give it too many fancy labels—colic, allergy, etc.—and don't treat it. Instead, understand it.

My baby is three months old and has just started to drool. Is he teething?

Contrary to popular belief, the onset of drooling is not usually associated with teething, which begins around five or six months of age. The salivary glands begin to function more actively at three to four months of age, which causes the drooling. Later, the infant becomes more adept at swallowing his saliva and the tendency to drool then disappears at around a year of age.

What can I do about spitting up?

Realize that it is a perfectly normal situation and that all babies will spit up from time to time. You may try the following: feed slowly, burp frequently, and avoid jostling him around immediately after the feeding. He will eventually outgrow the tendency as his nervous system matures and begins to suppress this undesirable reflex, usually by about eight months. In the meantime carry a towel and watch out if you are dressed up to go out and are feeding him in a hurry, for he will surely pick this time to perform!

My baby is colicky.

In the breast-fed baby the most frequent cause is something in the maternal diet that disagrees with him, as we have previously discussed. In the formula-fed baby, cow's milk allergy has to be at the top of the list. In infants who are on solid foods allergy is again a good bet and you may have to try an elimination diet to find the culprit. Then there are those infants who tend to be more gassy than others and eventually outgrow the tendency while parents and pediatrician exhaust themselves looking for a cause. Lastly there are some parents whose tolerance for what others might consider a normal amount of gassiness and colicky behavior is on the low side; a little understanding is what they need to get over the hump.

He is always chewing on things. Does that mean he is teething?

Yes, he probably is, but that's not the only reason he's always mouthing objects. Infants use oral exploration to gain information later obtained from hands, eyes, ears, and nose. These sensory areas are not as well developed at this age.

Do newborn babies breathe through the nose or mouth?

They are dependent on nose breathing, but in a very short time develop the neurological maturity to correlate mouth breathing and swallowing.

Sometimes he pulls at his ears. Is there something wrong with them?

Chances are there is nothing wrong unless he cries in discomfort or has signs of a cold. When tired, bored, or frustrated, babies of four to six months and occasionally older may pull at their ears. I suppose it is because they are so readily accessible and always available. Later on, they can chew on a pencil or perhaps put their glasses on and off!

I have noticed that since we have been home from the hospital he seems to sneeze and hiccup a lot. Is there anything I should do about it?

No. Sneezing and hiccuping are protective mechanisms which help clean his respiratory tract of any excess mucus after birth. These reflexes continue to be set off in little babies until about three or four months of age. At this time the nervous system has developed to a point where they are brought under better control.

At times his chin will quiver. Is this normal?

Yes. It is just a sign of immaturity of the nervous system. You will also notice that he occasionally is "jumpy" or startles, especially in response to loud noises or sudden movement.

How do you feel about pacifiers?

I don't like them but if you have a baby who simply seems to want to suck a great deal a pacifier isn't going to do any harm. In my experience the baby who is going to suck his thumb won't touch the pacifier. So don't think by forcing it on him you will prevent it. Popping in the "Binky" when junior hollers about anything is to me like popping in the tranquilizer as an adult. The instinctive desire to suck is present in infancy in order to ensure adequate nutrition. Later on one does not have to suck to eat and this means of satisfying hunger is dropped entirely. What you want to avoid as parents is prolonging sucking and using it to shut off unpleasant reactions in your child. It is far better to let him holler and perhaps find out why he's doing it than immediately to turn it off by the use of a conditioned response to an artificial "plug." Besides, he's got to learn to deal with frustration sooner or later.

How do I stop thumb-sucking?

Sucking is one of the strongest instinctual behavior patterns of the infant and is present from the moment of birth. There are great individual differences in the amount of sucking each infant requires. Furthermore, those who seem to enjoy sucking beyond the amount necessary to supply their nutritional needs will gravitate to the thumb since it is always readily available. The most important advice I can give is for parents to appreciate that this is an almost universal and normal phenomenon and that they should resist attempts to actively interfere with it since frequently they only add fuel to the fire. Pulling the thumb out of the mouth, putting on mittens, and annointing it with foul-tasting substances are all to be condemned. I've yet to see any college students who thumb-suck anyway.

ELIMINATION

Why does his urine smell like ammonia?

There's no mistaking that odor, is there? Don't worry, it is perfectly normal and comes from bacterial action on ammonia-containing compounds in the urine.

I have noticed that the diapers have a pink stain on them.

This rather faint pink color is from urate crystals, a normal constituent of the urine in early infancy.

What should his bowel movements look like and how often should he have them?

Breast-fed babies usually have frequent stools; every time you pick them up there's another one! Formula-fed babies usually have less frequent bowel movements. Those on whole milk vary, but on the whole this tends to constipate and thus the stools are usually firmer in consistency and less frequent. Usually the stool is a yellowish brown in the young infant and gradually darkens a bit as he gets older. Occasionally he may pass a greenish loose stool if something disagrees with him but this is usually a temporary situation. The breast-fed infant tends to have loose stools which appear somewhat pasty in consistency but as he gets older the general tendency is to firmer and less frequent bowel movements. Often by four to six months he may be having only two per day and this pattern may continue for quite some time. As he approaches his first birthday another change frequently takes place: the stools may become quite bulky, loose, and more frequent—three to five per day. I am sure that teething has some influence on this situation, but I also feel that the introduction of various foods also plays a role. This state may continue for several months and then gradually he will return to the previous pattern. I have followed many babies who do this and in some have tried various remedies such as allergy diets, gluten-free regimens, etc., none of which made the slightest difference. Throughout this period the baby continues to thrive while everyone frets over what to do about his BMs. In short, the answer is often nothing! The following may be of some help.

Frequency of BMs

BREAST-FED	FORMULA-FED
0–3 months: up to six to eight a day	every three to four days to three to four per day
3–6 months: three to four per day	one to three per day
6– same	six to twelve months: one to three per day twelve to eighteen months: one to four per day

To conclude this brief discussion of baby's BMs I would like to mention that as a general rule it is far more important to keep your eye on the baby and not on his stools. If there is something wrong it will reflect itself in the way he behaves.

My baby is constipated. What should I do?

There is almost never a call hour that does not contain at least one or two questions regarding constipation. I guess my approach to the matter is first of all to reassure the parents that for the most part this is not a serious matter, although it may be extremely distressing to both parent and patient.

First of all, let's find out if he is really constipated. To me the term *constipation* means the formation of stools which are hard enough in consistency to produce discomfort when they are passed. Usually the bowel movements are infrequent. I would like to stress that it is not the frequency but the fact that there is discomfort associated with the passage of the stool that is the most important factor in determining whether or not the baby is really constipated. This discomfort can occasionally be present when the stool does not appear to be that hard. A word of caution here— the production of a normal bowel movement requires a great deal of forceful muscular effort as well as complex reflex organization. Therefore an infant may turn red in the face, pass some gas, grunt, and yet pass a perfectly normal stool without any discomfort.

Now we come to one of the basic points of this whole business and that is the *wide* range of normality regarding the process of producing bowel movements. A breast-fed baby may have a stool following each nursing, six to ten per day, whereas one on formula may only produce one movement every three days, and yet both are happy and healthy. Even a breast-fed baby may only have a bowel movement once in twenty-four to forty-eight hours, although this is not the usual situation and most often lasts only for a short period of time. The differences in maternal diet may be a factor in this range of normality. One mother loves peaches, pears, prunes, and other laxative foods while the other eats apples, bananas, and drinks a great deal of milk, all of which tend to constipate. Then there is the difference in individual infants. Some absorb more water from the bowel than others and tend to have firmer and less frequent stools.

Now let's look at another factor—consistency. As you no doubt know, breast-fed babies tend to have looser stools than their formula-fed cohorts. That is not to say that the reverse cannot also be true, as previously mentioned. Let us suppose that a four-month-old baby on whole milk tends to have a firm stool. He passes this without difficulty. Is he constipated? No! Not unless someone says he is.

Most cases of constipation can easily be remedied by minor alterations in either the baby's or the mother's diet. Increasing the amount of fluid (other than milk, which often tends to constipate) and adding more laxative foods such as honey, apricots, and prunes usually corrects the situation promptly. I like to avoid using stool softeners in babies but occasionally adding a teaspoon of Karo syrup to one or two bottles of milk a day is helpful. On rare occasions the infant may become very uncomfortable and the stool almost rock hard. On these occasions an infant glycerine suppository may be used. More than an occasional use of a suppository is to be actively discouraged. Remember that an attack on the problem from the other end is far and away the better approach.

My major concern is that of overintervention. Don't start labeling a baby as constipated and use this term to explain a myriad of unrelated problems. Waking up in the middle of the night, changes in appetite, poor coloring, and a host of other difficulties are seldom due to constipation.

The emotional factors involved in bowel habits are of major significance and I want to emphasize that these factors come into play from the moment of birth. A relaxed and emotionally stable atmosphere results in the development of good bowel habits. A tense, unsettled environment, for reasons that are often remote from the infant, can produce serious problems. Start thinking of your baby as constipated and soon he may really be that way! Your anxieties over the bowel process, your and even your physician's overconcern with the number, frequency, and consistency of stools can lead not only to difficulty with toilet training, but also to a lifetime of problems with the process of elimination. Remember, the vast majority of constipated infants are healthy and thriving.

In conclusion keep in mind that this is a normal biological function with a wide range of normality and that it is *self*-regulating. Constant monitoring is therefore not required.

I noticed some blood in the baby's stools. What shall I do?

Usually this is red blood and coats the outside of the bowel movement. It most often results from the passage of a very hard stool, which has abraded some of the anal lining. Not only will it frequently cause some minor bleeding but more importantly these so-called anal fissures can produce a considerable amount of pain on defecation. Most of the time these small areas are not visible since they are just inside the anal opening.

Treatment consists in keeping the stools on the soft side for a few days until healing takes place. If this is not done then the infant may become severely constipated since the tendency is to withhold the stool because its passage is so painful.

In the breast-fed baby we occasionally encounter blood in the stool which emanates from a fissure or crack in the maternal nipple. In this case there is no discomfort on the part of the infant and the blood is usually intermixed with the stool. Often it is of a darker color, having been partially digested by the baby as it passes through the intestinal tract. Most often there is some maternal discomfort noted during nursing, although the actual bleeding point may not be seen. Usually the fissure results from excessive dryness of the skin or the nipple and is easily remedied by using one of the many creams available. Occasionally excessively prolonged or too frequent nursing can be a factor.

Will a change in water affect his stools?

Yes, it can, particularly if the change is to well water. Be sure that the well water has been checked for bacterial contamination when you go off to that summer place.

CLOTHING

How should I dress him?

In answer to this question I do not ever recall seeing a baby who was underdressed! I have, however, observed many who were sweating profusely and who otherwise manifested various signs of discomfort as they lay swaddled in all those goodies from baby showers plus the garments handed down or crocheted by Great-aunt Matilda. For many mothers I advise dressing the baby and then removing the top layer. A good rule to follow is to dress the baby in relation to what you are wearing.

What size clothes should I buy for the baby?

Make sure you buy those that are marked at least several months older than he is, for in my experience by the time you get them home and on him they are already too small!

How should I wash his clothes?

Your regular detergent should be all right, and no special additives, softeners, etc., are usually necessary.

KEEPING HIM HEALTHY AND CLEAN

How often should I take the baby to the doctor?

A good schedule is as follows:

> Once a month for the first six months
> Every two months for the second six months
> Every three months from one to two years
> Every six months from two to three years
> Once a year beginning at age three

I consider the monthly visit for the first six months to be vitally important for several reasons. First, during this time many treatable and correctable conditions can be detected—hearing loss, dislocation of the hip, and various forms of congenital heart disease, to name a few. Secondly, a great deal of valuable information regarding feeding, early development, and the like is given. Also, the basic immunizations are begun. Lastly, and of very great importance, this early period establishes a solid relationship between the parents and the pediatrician. The more they know about each other the more effectively they can work together in the challenge of child rearing.

Can I expect any reaction from his "baby" shot?

He will receive three primary shots of so-called DPT vaccine, at age two, four and six months, plus a booster at 18 months. DPT stands for diphtheria, pertussis (whooping cough), and tetanus. Frequently there is some degree of irritability and even a mild temperature of 101 to 102 rectal the late afternoon and evening following the shot. If this is the case you may give a dose of a single children's aspirin tablet (dissolve in water and give on the spoon). A high fever is more unusual (103 to 104) and should be reported to your doctor. Very often there is no fever but the infant reacts instead by becoming lethargic and sleeps soundly. Most reactions are over by the following morning and if fever persists you should check in. In my experience the second shot is far more likely to cause a reaction than the first or third. There is occasionally some redness at the injection site, and following the immunization there may be a firm nodular area deep in the muscle. This is formed by scar tissue and is of no consequence. In time it either goes away or is forgotten.

When and how often should I bathe him?

After the cord falls off and the area has healed you may bathe him: usually about ten days of age. I advise bathing twice to three times a week at most. Daily bathing has a drying effect on the skin; besides he usually isn't that dirty anyway. Midmorning is the best time as this is usually a calm period for both baby and mother.

He hates the bath

This happens frequently and usually occurs around six to eight months of age. Just sponge him lightly for a week or so, and his aversion to the bath will pass!

How shall I clean the ears?

Wax is a normal secretion of the ear canals. It protects and lubricates the lining and only rarely produces a problem of blockage in the older child and almost never in the baby. So don't be overzealous in cleaning it away. You may wipe gently with warm water around the external ear and even use a Q-tip in the skin folds but *do not* attempt to clean down in the ear canal. Not only is this a painful experience for the baby, but it is totally unnecessary and the delicate lining is easily irritated.

When and how should I cut the fingernails?

If he is scratching himself, and looks as though he has been in a fight, he needs them cut. Otherwise, they are just as well left alone and frequently they will break off themselves. To trim the nails, hold the hand firmly and always cut straight across.

I can see a hair in his eye. What shall I do to remove it?

Resist the temptation to remove it. It will gradually work its way out if given time to do so.

How do I clean my little girl's genitalia?

Use a washcloth dipped in plain water. Spread the labia gently and wipe downward gently once or twice. Do not use Q-tips.

What should I do about his navel? I have noticed several drops of blood.

Sponge the navel area lightly with rubbing alcohol once each day until the cord stump falls off. After the stump is off, the navel should be kept clean and dry with the use of some powder. During the time the cord stump is coming off there is frequently a small amount of bleeding for a few days. This is of no concern. As soon as the navel is healed the baby may be immersed in water for his first tub bath. This usually occurs around ten days of age.

I have noticed that his navel and attached cord have a distinct odor. Does this mean anything?

Yes, it means that the area is probably infected and you should call your physician. Normally the umbilicus is odorless.

How do I care for the circumcision?

The circumcision is performed usually one or two days before the baby leaves the hospital and takes four to five days to heal. A Vaseline gauze strip is applied immediately afterward to the open area. This prevents the exposed area from sticking to the diaper. Usually after 24 to 48 hours the penis may be left uncovered and no special care is required. During the healing process a whitish mucusy material forms over the glans. This is normal and does not represent infection. The tip (glans) of the penis frequently has a purplish color, also normal. After healing, regular soap and water may be used. Remember to retract the foreskin daily so that adhesions do not take place. Your doctor will show you how.

Should I take the baby's temperature routinely?

There is no need to take his temperature on a routine basis. If he is acting sick in some way, then it's a good idea to check. The normal rectal temperature is approximately one degree higher (99 to 100°) than the oral temperature.

My baby is only two months old and has a temperature of 102. I have heard that this is more serious in a small baby. Is this true?

Yes, fever is an infant three months or less can mean a serious illness, and you should check in with your doctor immediately.

SKIN

What can I do for a diaper rash?

A few good rules:

Change frequently.

Don't use rubber pants early. Most babies do not tolerate them until four to five months of age and even then it is wise to discontinue them temporarily at the first sign of a rash.

Disposable diapers are great! The only trouble is that they are sometimes too good. Not only are they very absorbent, but they fit very snugly and do not allow enough air to circulate, therefore setting the stage for a good old diaper rash. By all means use them, but at the first sign of skin irritation go back to the old-fashioned baggy but effective, loose-fitting cotton diaper. An occasional infant does not tolerate them at all, but fortunately for parents this is not a frequent situation.

Exposing the diaper area to the air is the most important factor—even though with little boys you run the risk of getting an unexpected dousing! Still, clean, dry skin is your best means of prevention as well as most important treatment.

Resist the temptation to anoint the baby with creams or powders. If your aesthetic sensibilities dictate the use of something, then try a *small* amount of baby powder after each change, but rub it in well. Caking on a nice heavy layer may make you feel good but it will effectively block the skin pores and frequently produce the very rash you are trying so assiduously to prevent. All in all, a mild soap such as castile and plain water are by far your best allies.

Don't feel that you are a failure if a rash develops. All babies develop one at some point. Never a week goes by that a mother or father does not appear in the office, reluctant to remove the diaper for a well-baby examination. Immediately I know that underneath a rash is waiting.

There are numerous powders and ointments that can be used for established rashes. Your doctor will tell you his favorite. Dietary factors are an important cause. Lots of juice, especially orange and apple, as well as many other fruits, can produce skin irritation. Occasionally a vitamin drop preparation can cause difficulty. Remember, *clean* and *dry* are the watchwords.

Are disposable wipes all right to use on the baby? We find that they are very convenient when we are out somewhere and he needs changing?
They are perfectly all right to use.

When can I use rubber pants?
By three to four months of age. If used earlier you may produce a diaper rash by the combination of sensitive skin and lack of sufficient aeration.

What is prickly heat?
This is a fine, reddish, bumpy rash that is produced by the blockage of small sweat and sebaceous glands in the skin. No creams or powders are needed; in fact they may aggravate the condition by further blocking the skin pores. To clear it up dress him lightly and allow air to get to the skin.

My baby has thrush. Is it serious and what should be done about it?
Thrush is caused by a yeast and is frequent in infants. It is rarely serious and usually occurs in the mouth or diaper area. Your doctor will prescribe medication which should clear it up promptly. Vaginal infections in the mother are the most frequent source. In addition it can be transmitted via the maternal nipple in breast-fed babies, and also to bottle-fed babies through a nipple that has not been cleaned properly. Incidental skin infection in the mother is occasionally a cause.

What can you tell me about birthmarks on the skin?
Babies are often born with localized areas of pinkish pigmentation of the skin. They most frequently occur over the eyelids and at the back of the neck. These are completely innocuous

and will almost always disappear by the end of the first year. They are often referred to as stork bites. Other marks have a deep strawberry color and appearance and are often raised from the surface of the skin. These are made of small groups of blood vessels. They are almost invariably benign and will most often fade away if given sufficient time, although sometimes this may take several years.

What causes the bumpy rash on his face?

Frequently babies develop a rash characterized by reddish "bumps" usually located on the cheeks and chin. This rash is due to blockage of the pores of little sweat and sebaceous glands in the skin, and is often associated with rubbing the face against the sheet or blanket, drooling, and by the accumulation of solid food, most frequently cereal, over the area during feeding. No specific treatment is necessary and the rash usually comes and goes on its own. It never bothers the baby so don't let it bother you! Gradually he will outgrow it anyway.

What is cradle cap?

A scaly, bumpy rash over the scalp is referred to as cradle cap because in severe cases it appears in a caplike distribution. It is caused by overexuberant sweat and sebaceous glands that secrete an excess of skin oil. It tends to run in families. Other areas frequently affected include the skin behind the ears, the ear canals, the eyelids, and the skin folds of the groin and under the arms. Most infants will outgrow their problem at about six to eight months of age but in some it may persist. It is one of the causes of dandruff in the adult. Cradle cap most often appears at three to six weeks of age. Heat, as it results in increased sweating, will aggravate the condition. Treatment consists of brushing away the scales on the scalp and rubbing in some regular olive oil two to three times a week. If this is not helpful then a special antiseborrhea shampoo may do the job. Occasionally the rash becomes more generalized over the body, which may be due to food allergies.

The baby's skin is peeling. What should I do about it?

Nothing. Shortly after birth there is frequently some flaking off of the skin over various parts of the body. It is often most pronounced over the hands and feet and may continue for one or two weeks. This normal process requires no special care. In fact, a good general rule is to resist the strong desire to oil, cream, powder, and otherwise minister to the skin.

I can see several bluish areas under the baby's skin, especially on the forehead and around the nose. What are they?

These are veins. A baby's skin is quite translucent due to the absence of a good deal of subcutaneous tissue. As he gets older you won't be able to see them.

I notice that my baby's skin gets a "blotchy" bluish-purplish color when he is undressed.

This mottling of the skin is quite frequent in babies when they are exposed to cool air and immediately disappears as the baby is warmed. This may occur in older children and adults as well but is more pronounced in infants because of the immaturity in controlling the blood flow in the skin. The same phenomenon produces the blue hands and feet so often seen. In any case it is no cause for concern.

TEETH

What should I do about teething?

Generally, you won't have to do a thing. With all the terrible things attributed to teething many mothers wonder if they will be able to survive the ordeal. Believe it or not, most babies and parents have no difficulty at all. Occasionally an aspirin helps, and a bit of bourbon rubbed on the gums is all right too. A moderate degree of fussiness, some loosening and increased frequency of the stools, and diaper rashes all are more likely to occur at this time. Drooling and a mild degree of nasal congestion are sometimes present. I do not think that teething produces fever, but not all pediatricians agree.

The first teeth usually appear at around six months of age.

Can you tell me what teeth to expect when?

The deciduous or primary teeth erupt as follows:

Two lower central incisors, 5 to 7 months
Four upper central incisors, 7 to 8 months
Two lower lateral incisors, 8 to 12 months
Four first-year molars, 10 to 16 months
Four canine teeth, 16 to 20 months
Four second-year molars, 20 to 30 months

In my experience teething patterns vary a great deal, both as to time and sequence of eruption. Babies don't read the books! It is not infrequent for the first tooth to appear as late as a year of age. Family history is an important factor. It is not true that if the teeth erupt early they will not be good teeth.

It has always been a source of fascination to me why so much emphasis is placed on teeth and the time of their appearance. The time of eruption and sequence do not correlate with any phase of development, either intellectually or other, of which I am aware, yet they remain a source of unending interest to most all parents.

My one-year-old has two bluish swollen areas on the gums. Are they blood clots or something?

As the teeth erupt, particularly the molars, there is frequently some entrapped blood over the top of the tooth. This is no cause for concern. There may even be some bleeding as the tooth erupts, but it is almost always swallowed immediately and so you are not even aware of it.

There is a gap between his teeth. Will it go away?

The baby teeth are frequently widely separated. This is especially true of the upper central incisors. In addition they may appear angulated or rotated. By the time all the baby teeth are in place they are almost always properly aligned.

What should be done about a tooth that is present at birth?

If the natal tooth is firmly in place then nothing need be done. If it is loose it should be removed, as there is a danger of swallowing it. It may also have to be removed if it bothers the nursing mother. These teeth are usually primary teeth that have erupted too soon, and many have incomplete root structures. It will not be replaced until the permanent teeth come in. If the tooth is a supernumerary or extra tooth it may be removed. An X ray is the only way to be sure which type it is.

I am breast-feeding my baby. Do I need to give him fluoride?

Even though a negligible amount of fluoride comes through in the breast milk he doesn't need any fluoride supplementation until after six months of age and only then if he is not getting occasional fluoridated water or fluoride from various solid foods, or if you live in an area where the water does not contain sufficient amounts of fluoride. Thus children living in areas with fluoridated water do not require supplemental doses. However, fluorides may be prescribed later if he shows a marked tendency to caries formation. An occasional bottle of water given to the breast-fed infant would seem to be sufficient to meet fluoride requirements in that age group.

EYES

When can he see?

A newborn baby will blink in response to a bright light and will even fixate briefly on a red ring of about three inches in diameter. Babies in the nursery will tend to turn toward a light source. At approximately six weeks of age he develops a social smile upon seeing mother and by three months of age he will follow an object or person through a 180 degree arc. The capacity to assign meaning to what is seen develops throughout the period of infancy and beyond.

My baby's eyes are red and swollen shut. Is something wrong?

Most likely not. This is a normal "chemical conjunctivitis" caused by silver nitrate drops that are put in the baby's eyes at birth in order to prevent gonorrhea of the eye, which used to be among the leading causes of blindness. It will all clear up promptly, usually within 24 to 48 hours.

What does it mean when he squints his eyes in the sun?
It means that he is behaving quite normally.

I have noticed that one pupil seems larger than the other. Is this serious?
Your doctor will want to check this out but he probably has a condition where there is a disparity in pupil size from birth. This causes no problems and is of no concern other than noting its existence. The only reason to be aware of it is that one of the classic danger signs following head injury is the development of unequal pupils, so it is wise to know whether or not your child has always been that way.

I've noticed that the white part of his eye has a bluish tint. Is that normal?
Yes, it is. The sclera or white of the eye normally has a slight bluish coloration in the infant. This gradually changes to a white color with age. There is a genetic abnormality where the sclera is often quite blue at birth and remains so throughout life but this is extremely rare.

Can the eyes appear crossed and yet really not be?
Yes. Frequently an illusion of crossed eyes is produced by the asymmetry of the skin folds on the inner corner of the eye. These folds are often prominent in little babies and if one is larger than the other it will cover more of the white of the eye or sclera on that side and make it appear that the eye is deviating inwardly, especially when the infant looks to one side. As he grows older these folds gradually recede. If one shines a light into the eyes it will be reflected in both pupils or dark spots in exactly the same place. It is these same epicanthic folds which persist in Orientals and give the illusion of slanting eyes.

When will his eyes change color?
All infants are born with blue eyes. If they are going to change color they will usually begin to do so by three to four months of age. Occasionally a color change may occur as late as 10 to 12 months.

There is a blood spot in the eye. Will it need treatment and what causes it?

Anything that raises pressure within the eye can cause a small blood vessel in the inside of the eye to rupture and bleed. The normal passage through the birth canal often produces this kind of pressure, as can forceful coughing, sneezing, and vomiting. These hemorrhages resolve spontaneously and although they may frighten you, they result in no damage to the eye.

When will he develop tears?

Tears are present at birth and are constantly needed to protect the eye from harmful drying effects. These tears are small in quantity and originate from small glands along the eyelids. They are usually not noted, however, until they begin to overflow the eyelids, which usually occurs either early in infancy because of a blocked tear duct, or until reflex production of tears from the lacrimal gland in response to crying or discomfort begins at approximately three months of age. Before this time he may be howling mad but there is not a tear in sight.

When does binocular vision develop?

As early as six months of age the infant can be shown to have good depth perception and therefore binocular vision.

My baby has something wrong with his eye. It is always "runny." What can I do?

In order to understand what may appear to be excess moisture in the eye I must give a brief explanation of the tear mechanism. Tears are produced by small glands in the eyelids. The tears then flow across the eye toward the nose and go into a small opening and from there into a small tube or duct which empties into the nose. If, as is often the case, this duct is not open, or if it is only partially open, as is the usual case, the tears will "back up" in the eye and overflow onto the cheek. This gives the eye a wet appearance and there is often excessive "mattering" or "sleep" in the eye. Wiping the eye with a clean washcloth will help to reduce crusting, and I think that it is a good idea to massage the lacrimal sac several times a day to help open the duct, which is directly underneath. Let your physician show you this simple maneuver. Incidentally, massaging down the side of the nose, as is frequently taught, has no effect on the duct since it does not lie in this area. Most of the time the duct will open spontaneously by five to six months of age. If it has not, or if there has been infection present, then the ophthalmologist may need to insert a small probe to open it. This procedure can be done in his office. If not taken care of in infancy this easily correctable condition can lead to permanent scarring of the tear duct, which will require extensive surgical correction.

Is it permissible to use flashbulbs to take his picture?

Yes, indeed. His protective blink reflex is well developed at birth and bright light will not hurt him.

See Chapter 9 for more on the subject of eyes and vision.

LEGS AND FEET

His feet are flat.

They are supposed to be. There is a good deal of fatty tissue on the sole of the foot which makes it devoid of any arch. As he begins to walk the arch will gradually develop.

He has bow legs!

You are right! They are supposed to be that way and gradually will straighten as he grows older. Early walkers have more of this condition than late walkers. This cowboy appearance reaches its zenith at about 16 to 20 months of age and then gradually *self-corrects*. In almost all cases it requires no treatment, but occasionally your doctor may advise a splint of some kind for a short time.

One foot seems to turn in more than the other.

This condition, termed "windblown feet," is frequently seen as the infant begins to walk and usually self-corrects within a few weeks.

I have noticed that his toes overlap. Is this a condition that needs correction?

Overlapping of the toes, usually the third and fourth toe, is seen fairly often in infants and is of no significance. It often runs in families.

My baby's feet turn out. Is there something wrong?

Babies with feet that turn outward usually have nothing wrong at all and the feet will eventually straighten out, but usually not until he walks. Infants with feet that turn out are often a bit slower to walk than others, perhaps because of the forward-and-backward balance problem created by the foot in this position.

His feet turn in.

This is true in almost all babies. For the first few weeks he can easily be folded back into the fetal position. In this posture his legs are bowed and the feet are inwardly rotated. Occasionally the front of the foot turns in rather sharply and in this condition your doctor may prescribe an "outflare" shoe for the baby that will usually correct the problem in a few weeks. In time spontaneous derotation takes place in the majority of cases. A tendency to toe in may persist and most of the time requires no treatment. Quite to the contrary, since the majority of good athletes toe in. So take heart—instead of having an orthopedic problem he may be heading for an athletic scholarship.

Can you tell me something about dislocation of the hip?

Congenital hip dislocation occurs more frequently in girls and is essentially a condition where the hip socket is rather shallow and the head of the thighbone is not inside the socket. Most of the time it occurs on only one side but occasionally both hips are involved. Some signs of its presence are tightness in spreading the hips, shortening of one leg, and an asymmetric appearance of the legs or feet. Asymmetry of the skin folds (different appearance on the two sides) is seen frequently in little babies and generally means nothing, if not associated with some other finding. With a mild congenital hip problem there is no dislocation, only minimal muscle tightness. It is important to remember that this is a condition that has an excellent prognosis if diagnosed early and it is therefore of utmost importance that your baby's hips be carefully checked on each visit to your doctor.

Will standing up bow his legs?

No, but not allowing him to do it will deprive him of a lot of fun. Babies who walk at an early age tend to have more bowing than those who walk at a later age. It is of no concern, however, since the legs will almost always undergo gradual straightening as he gets older.

When does he need his first pair of shoes?

Not until he is beginning to walk. Save your money and don't buy them any earlier. He doesn't need them to shape his foot, help him learn to walk, or for any other reason than warmth and protection of the foot. Going barefoot is an excellent idea wherever practical.

What type of shoes should I buy? Must they be high-topped?

High-topped shoes are not necessary at all and your baby can start off with any type of shoe. This may be heresy but it's true, nevertheless. Whether or not he is going to be flat-footed is determined genetically and not by the shoes he wears. In addition they need not be white. Any shoe that fits and any color you can live with!

EARS

When does he hear?

A baby's hearing is acute at birth. In the first few months of life he will startle (give a big jump) at a sudden loud noise. In most infants this gradually lessens at about six months of age but can persist longer. An infant will localize sound at approximately six to seven months and will turn his head in the direction from which the sound emanates. Sometimes a baby will not respond to certain noises. One may need to try a wide range of sounds (rattling keys, crinkling paper, tapping wooden blocks, ringing a small bell) in order to see a response. If, on several occasions, no response is obtained, one should be concerned. The most important factor in the early detection of hearing deficits in infants is the observation of the parents, so take careful note. Babies with severe hearing loss usually are quieter in general and do not develop the wide range of babbling, cooing, and jargon of the normal infant. Bring up any question you have with your doctor since early detection is important. Audiological techniques for the accurate evaluation of hearing loss in infants are well developed and, if necessary, hearing aids can be applied under a year of age.

What is the incidence of hearing impairment in babies?

Approximately 1 in 1200 babies will turn out to have some degree of hearing impairment at birth. Between birth and five years of age another 6 to 7 per 1200 will be diagnosed to run the total to 7 to 8 children per 1200.

Are there any risk factors for hearing loss to be aware of?

Any of the following will put your baby in the high-risk category for possible hearing loss:

Family history of hearing loss from early life

Premature birth

Any baby who has had an elevation of bilirubin (jaundice) or who has required care in the intensive-care nursery

History of German measles during pregnancy or other viral infections in the first trimester

Obvious physical deformities of the ear

How early can you tell that the hearing is impaired?

Within a few days of birth one can begin to get an idea if the baby hears and serial (consecutive) observations by a trained observer should be made if there is continuing doubt about a baby's hearing. Arousal from light sleep by a noise is a particularly important indication that your baby hears normally, as is his response to the spoken voice and other noises and his startle response to loud noise.

Is it important to make the diagnosis of hearing impairment as soon as possible?

Yes, it certainly is, since even in the first few weeks of life the infant is already embarking on language development by selecting and patterning responses to sound.

Are there any specialized tests of hearing function that can be performed early in infancy to evaluate the baby's hearing?

Yes, several relatively new and sophisticated electrical devices measure a baby's hearing within even the first six months of life, but they are not always reliable and their results therefore must be interpreted cautiously.

What are some early signs that my baby's hearing is OK?

In the first two months he will startle to noise from a light sleep state.

By three months he will orient to familiar sounds, especially mother's voice.

By three to five months he will stop what he is doing momentarily in response to mother's voice, softly spoken.

By eight months a baby will localize sound—look in the direction of the sound.

At what age can a hearing aid be used?

As early as five to six months of age. The earlier you introduce amplified sound to a baby with hearing impairment, the better it is for language development.

Is there any way to stimulate good language development?

The baby acquires language by learning from the environment, most particularly from the mother. So it is important to talk with your baby from day one and to react to his verbalization.

Sometimes the baby has jumpy or jittery movements.

Most babies have some degree of tremulousness at times, either when startled or often when they are crying hard. This gradually diminishes by three to four months of age, as the nervous system matures.

For more about the evaluation of hearing see the beginning of Chapter 8.

There is a tiny hole in front of his ear.

Chances are it will never give him any trouble so there is no need to tamper with it. There is a small possibility that later it might become infected; if it does it is simple to remove.

His ears stick way out.

Occasionally the ear may be missing one of the normal cartilaginous folds and protrude in Dumbo-like fashion. We call it a lop ear. This can be a source of considerable embarrassment to the older child and adult and can be corrected in the school-age child by a simple surgical procedure done by the plastic surgeon. At birth the baby's ears may be excessively flattened, bent over, and otherwise pushed out of shape but given a little time they unfold nicely.

My baby's ear is folded over. What can I do about it?

Nothing needs to be done. It is due to his position in the uterus and will straight out spontaneously in a very short time, most often in a matter of days.

HEAD

His head is such a funny shape.

There is a good deal of molding of the head that takes place as the baby comes through the birth canal, so that a newborn's head often appears elongated and "banana shaped." This will gradually self-correct. Occasionally one sees a large swelling toward the back of the head, on one or both sides. It may be barely noticeable until the second or third day of life and may take several months to gradually be absorbed.

My baby has a large lump on the back of his head. My pediatrician gave it a long name and said it would go away. What do you think?

It is probably a cephalohematoma, which is a collection of blood under the scalp but *outside* the skull which is produced, not infrequently, by the rupture of small blood vessels under the scalp as the baby's head passes through the birth canal. It may not be apparent until several days after birth; eventually the blood is reabsorbed and it will go away spontaneously over the ensuing weeks or months.

Why does he have a soft spot?

The skull of a baby is made up of several bones. Where two bones are adjacent to one another there is a linear opening. Where more than two bones join there are soft spots. One of them is in the back of the head and usually closes at about six weeks of age. The other is on top of the head toward the front. This may stay open up to 18 months of age and in some cases even longer. These spaces are open in order to accommodate brain growth.

Can I brush over the soft spot? How soft is it anyway?

Let's answer the second part first. The soft spot is really a misnomer. This area is covered by a membrane that is as tough as thick canvas and just as protective as the skull bones. So the answer to your first question is obvious.

Is there any significance to the size of the soft spot?

No. As long as it is open and does not close prematurely. Your doctor will check it regularly and take head measurements to make sure that the head is growing at a normal rate.

I have noticed that the baby's soft spot pulsates. Is this normal?

Yes, it is. The pulsation of the blood vessels in the brain is transmitted through the fluid over the surface and can be distinctly felt in many babies and seen as well. It is also normal that no pulsation is felt as the baby gets a bit older, about five to six months.

My baby seems to keep his head to one side a great deal of the time. Is there something wrong?

Yes, he probably has a condition in which one of the neck muscles is tight. Your doctor will instruct you in exercises that will take care of the problem.

COUGHING, SNEEZING, AND COLDS

When is he likely to catch his first cold?

Usually at about five to six months of age. It is at this time that the antibodies which you gave him during pregnancy begin to disappear and his own production is getting started. If he is a first baby the first cold may not appear until much later. If he is a member of a rapidly growing family, chances are that he will be exposed by his siblings at an earlier date.

He has started to cough at various times and yet he seems to feel fine.

I am frequently asked this question about an infant who is four to five months of age. Most often he isn't sick and your observations are entirely correct. He has learned how to cough and has added this sound to his verbal repertoire. Often you will notice he will give a big smile of satisfaction after he finishes.

He has a stuffy nose all the time. Is it a cold?

Usually not. A baby's nasal passages are smaller in proportion to the remainder of his airway than an adult's and his breathing therefore tends to be noisier. Also he may be suffering from being raised in our affluent society, a victim of central heating and air conditioning. Both reduce the humidity to very low levels. This acts to irritate the respiratory tract and often produces nasal congestion and "noisy breathing." A central humidifier is a great help, as is a cold-steam vaporizer run in the room at night. This is good for parents as well as the baby. Persistent nasal congestion in a baby who does not act ill is often a sign of allergy that may well need to be explored. Allergic symptoms can appear at a very early age. They may be caused by foods but also inhalants such as house dust, mold, and animal dander.

What kind of cough medicine can be given to a baby?

You should check with the pediatrician about the nature of the cough before administering any medication. If a cough medicine is needed for a baby under a year of age, the following is a good one. Mix one ounce of honey with an ounce of lemon juice and add two teaspoons of bourbon (or Scotch if you prefer) to top it off. One teaspoon of this may be given every four to six hours.

MORE ABOUT HIS BODY

What is tongue-tie and what should be done about it?

This is where the piece of skin under the front of the tongue, called the frenulum, is quite short, prevents normal tongue movement, and interferes with speech. To check, see if the child can touch the roof of his mouth with the tip of his tongue or if he can stick his tongue out over his lip. When the frenulum is too tight a simple surgical procedure is necessary, but most of the time the condition requires no treatment.

What is meant by a sunken chest?

Many infants have a tendency toward an indented breastbone and only rarely is it of any concern.

My baby seems to have such a long torso. Is this normal?

Yes, it is. Babies tend to have a much longer trunk in proportion to their arms and legs than do older children and adults.

His ribs stick out. Is this OK?

There is often some "flaring out" of the lower part of the rib cage and this is perfectly normal.

I notice a dimple at the base of the spine. What is it?

These are quite common and usually cause no trouble. Occasionally there is a small hole in the middle of the indentation that is called a sinus. In some cases this may communicate with a small cyst at its base. Rarely this becomes swollen and tender due to infection. When this occurs it is usually in the adolescent or adult age group.

He seems to have a couple of "funny-looking" skin folds near the base of his spine.

Frequently the skin folds here are not symmetrical and may tend to be much more pronounced in one direction or the other.

It makes no difference. In a baby this area is indeed very noticeable but later on it becomes one of the least noticed parts of the entire anatomy.

He has a bluish area near the base of his spine. What is it?

It is an area where the blood vessels are dilated and called a Mongolian spot. These bluish birthmarks can be quite large and most often occur over the lower back and buttocks. They are frequent in black and Oriental babies. They will go away, so don't be concerned.

What causes vaginal bleeding in the newborn?

Maternal hormones that have crossed the placenta during pregnancy. The amount of bleeding is small and usually ceases in a few days.

My baby had an erection. Is this normal?

Yes, erections in infancy are common and normal in boy babies.

I notice that every now and then when I move the baby's arm or leg there is a clicking sound. Is there something wrong?

This is a frequent observation. The clicking sound is usually made by a tendon gliding over the bone as the extremity is moved and is of no significance.

My baby has some bumps on his gums. What are they?

These are called retention cysts or pearls and are quite common along the gum margins. Small white cysts may also appear on the roof of the mouth. These are called Epstein's pearls because of their white shiny appearance. All of these are normal and will spontaneously disappear in time.

There seems to be a cyst or something on his lips.

These areas are produced by vigorous sucking, which goes to show you that you have a nice, healthy baby.

His tummy sticks way out to the side. Is this normal?

Yes. This is because the abdominal muscles are not as yet developed to the point where they will hold him in. His configuration is considerably different from that of the adult—big head, relatively short arms and legs as compared to trunk, and considerably more tummy than chest.

My baby seems to have a bulge, like a line down the middle of his stomach. It's not there all the time.

What you are seeing is the space between the two large abdominal muscles. When he cries or strains you may notice some bulging in this area but it is nothing to worry about, and as the rest of his abdominal muscles get stronger it will no longer be visible.

There is a bump that I can feel at the upper part of his tummy.

Right you are. This little protuberance is at the very tip of the breastbone. It is somewhat soft because it is made of cartilage and is movable. It goes by the fascinating name of the xyphoid process. You might use this in your next game of Scrabble.

My baby is very hairy.

Many babies, especially dark-skinned brunettes, have quite a bit of hair over the body as well as the arms and legs. This will gradually fall out over a period of several months.

His umbilicus seems to protrude. Is there anything we can do about it?

Some heal in, the others slightly out, and when not associated with a hernia there is no need to do anything at all. In time it usually tucks in a bit.

The doctor says that my baby has an accessory nipple. What is it?

An accessory nipple is a nipple in addition to the two normal ones. It may be located anywhere along the so-called milk line, the line that runs down the front of the body from the nipple. Although most of the time they occur on only one side and are single, they may occasionally occur on both sides and be multiple. They remain as they are and nothing need be done. Very unusually there may be associated breast tissue, and some type of cosmetic surgery may be required if an accessory breast should develop.

My baby has inverted nipples. Is there something that should be done about them?

No, nothing need be done, but you should expect them to remain that way. If the baby is a girl there is no reason why she will not be able to nurse her offspring someday, so there is no cause for concern.

Is it all right if the breasts are enlarged?

Yes, the enlargement of the breasts occurs frequently in both girl and boy babies. Maternal hormones cross the placenta during pregnancy and have a stimulating effect on the breast tissue. The swelling can be quite pronounced, is not tender, and produces no discomfort. It usually pretty well recedes by three months of age.

He has ingrown toenails.

They often appear that way, especially in the newborn period, but rarely do they cause any difficulty. Leave them alone!

I notice that he sweats a lot. Is there something wrong?

There is a considerable amount of variation in the amount of infant sweating, just as there is in children and adults. I think of several of my friends who, after playing two sets of tennis on a hot day, are perfectly dry while I stand there dripping!

My doctor discovered that my baby had a hernia. What is it and what should be done about it?

There are several different types of hernias. The umbilical hernia which is the one that produces a bulge at the navel area (umbilicus) is very common, is more frequent in black babies, and usually goes away on its own if left alone. The use of coins, bandages and other devices is to be discouraged since they may irritate the skin, prove a challenge to keep in place, inhibit good muscle development, and are unsightly as well.

The inguinal hernia is one that occurs more frequently in boys and is located in the groin. It usually is first noted as a bulge, which may extend down into the scrotum on the affected side or sides. Often the bulge is first noted when the infant or child cries or otherwise strains. These maneuvers increase the pressure inside the abdomen and force some of the abdominal contents outward through the so-called inguinal ring, which produces the bulge. Almost always the contents slide back inside the abdomen without difficulty and there are no symptoms related to the hernia. If the bulge seems to persist, then placing the infant in a reclining position and getting him as relaxed as possible will, along with gentle pressure on the hernia contents, "reduce" the hernia (that is, cause the herniated contents to slide back inside the abdomen). If the hernia cannot be reduced in a few minutes and becomes "stuck," we call it *incarcerated*; then something must be done about it immediately. It will soon produce pain and can lead to serious consequences. It is a genuine surgical emergency and if your doctor cannot be reached immediately then you should take your child to the hospital.

Most of the time inguinal hernias are discovered by the parents, and often the doctor does not actually see the hernia in the office but may confirm it on his examination. All inguinal hernias need to be surgically repaired, but can be done electively at a convenient time and are not emergencies (except when and if they become incarcerated). Because so many of them occur on both sides (bilateral), the feeling is that both sides sould be repaired at the time of surgery even though a bulge has been noted only on one side. It is a relatively simple operative procedure and the infant and young child tolerate it very well. Usually it requires merely an overnight stay in the hospital and the resultant scar can barely be noticed, as no external stitches are even used.

My six-week-old baby was just diagnosed as having pyloric stenosis. Can you tell me something about this condition?

It is caused by a thickening of the muscle that lines the stomach. This thickening can actually be enough to block the outlet portion of the stomach and therefore results in vomiting that is usually very forceful and is called *projectile vomiting*. It may actually shoot out three to four feet, so it's much different than the spitting up that babies frequently do. This condition is most common in firstborn male babies and the cause is unknown, although it may frequently run in families. The treatment is usually a simple surgical procedure to cut through this thickened band of muscle. This usually requires a hospital stay of three or four days. The usual age for pyloric stenosis to develop is about four to six weeks.

There is a small piece of skin near the anal area. Is it a hemorrhoid?

Frequently there are small tissue tags in the perianal area. They do no harm and nothing need be done about them.

I noticed that my one-year-old had a small bulge near the anal area that looked sort of purplish in color. Sometimes I see it, but at other times it is not there. I wonder if it is a hemorrhoid?

I have never seen a hemorrhoid in childhood, and although you are always taught never to say never in medicine you can almost do it in this case. Chances are what you are seeing is a piece of the anal mucosa or lining that occasionally may protrude a bit, but this is of no significance.

Is there any known cause for crib death?

There is still no known cause. A collaborative nationwide study is in process and, we hope, will provide us the answer to the number one killer of infants in the early months of life.

Growth and Development

Recently I have read a good deal about different personality types and different developmental patterns. Is there anything to it?

In the past we have come down a bit heavily on the side of the environment. So much of what the infant or child did or did not do was attributed to the parents or others dealing with him. Now, much more evidence indicates that the baby arrives on the scene with a great deal of his personality and intellectual potential already developed. One can recognize the tense, high-strung infant in contrast to the more placid one. The active little guy who is always on the go is the one who takes four people to hold him long enough to get him dressed after the pediatrician has examined him. In order to be successful parents, much of what we do must be based on a good understanding of the genetic constitution of our offspring, not only their IQs, but more importantly, their personality patterns. Failure to understand and indeed even to look at this aspect of child rearing is responsible for many problems later on. Blaming yourselves for your child's difficult behavior rather than understanding that you may have a difficult child is an all-too-common pitfall in child rearing. Furthermore, we are frequently so busy trying to mold the child to fit our expectations that we often do not take the time to understand him as an individual. The recognition and understanding of these inherent differences can be the source of as much or more enjoyment than similarities.

Are there any good ways of predicting growth?
Family history is most important. Otherwise, in girls we double the height at 18 months and can come up with a pretty good estimate. For boys, double at age two years. Although this is a fairly good general rule it may not apply to your child, so don't get hung up on it.

Is there any correlation between birth weight and ultimate size?
No, there is not. Family history of size does, however, correlate well with ultimate height.

What about length of the baby? Is this a good indicator of how tall he will be?
Yes, there is good correlation, but one word of caution here. Most babies have a good deal of flexor tone; that is, their legs are bent up the way they were positioned in the uterus, and this makes any accurate measurement of length at birth very difficult.

When should the baby double his birth weight?
At about four months of age.

How much does a baby grow in the first year?
An extraordinary amount! Approximately one inch and one and a half pounds per month for the first four to five months.

This rate is roughly halved in the second six months and further decreases during the second year of life.

At what age does hand preference usually develop?

Usually by one year of age some hand preference is discernible, although further delay in establishing laterality is no cause for concern and no attempt should be made to influence its development.

What can I do to stimulate his development?

The best way is to provide a stable, loving, caring environment, then relax and enjoy seeing him develop spontaneously! There is no need for gimmicks to help him, such as devices to help him crawl at an earlier date or swim before his first birthday. They not only don't work but they often alter the spontaneous path of normal development. Avoid overstimulation, which can be harmful because it adds stress and anxiety to the child-rearing process.

Are there any exercises that I should do with the baby?

Take a few minutes and just watch your baby. The amount of muscular effort he puts forth in a few minutes is astounding. Even a newborn can lie prone with his chin and feet off the ground—you try it! No, he certainly doesn't need any exercise program but you might!

If my child never goes through a crawling stage will it mean that he will have difficulty with reading later on?

Although the "normal" developmental pattern described in books is sitting, crawling, pulling to standing, and walking, a surprising number do not appear to have read this and skip the crawling stage altogether. Instead they pull to standing and once they have taken a few steps they are not about to go back to crawling. As far as I am concerned there is not one whit of evidence that these babies will have any more educational difficulties than their peers.

How do you feel about infant swimming?

Despite all the hoopla recently it is rare to find a child under two years of age who can swim unsupported in the water. They may have a wonderful time trying, but few ever seem to be successful. Therefore if you approach this whole business with the idea that it is going to be fun for both mother and infant to attend some regular swimming classes, then I am all for it. Just don't be disappointed or feel that you both are failures if he isn't ready for the swimming team when you finish.

Do you approve of a playpen?

Yes, indeed. Safety dictates that an infant who is into the crawling stage must have some restriction; otherwise you will not be able to leave him even momentarily. I have heard it said that looking through a mesh playpen will cause the eyes to cross—don't believe it!

My ten-month-old heads for my favorite vase in the living room. What can I do about it?

I would tell him no in such a way that you are sure he fully understands. If he still goes for it then he gets banished to his room for 20 to 30 minutes. It's important to understand that infants of this age, and even a good deal younger, understand at least three times as much as any of us, and that includes many physicians, give them credit for. There should be no need to strip the house bare. You are building up a relationship where he is going to follow your instructions. Later it will be "don't cross that street" and later still "be home by ten o'clock."

His Environment

I'm planning to go back to work. How old should the baby be when I do this and will my absence harm him?

I think that six to eight weeks (and preferably eight) is about the earliest a mother should return to a full-time job. The percentage of mothers who work has skyrocketed in the past few years and from my observations I am not aware that this has been the cause of any great increase in emotional problems. At all stages of child development it is not the *quantity* of time spent together but the *quality* that really makes the difference. A mother who wants to work but is staying home out of fear that working will harm her baby's emotional development is probably doing harm to the baby as well as herself. If she is happy, the baby will reap the positive input. Of course, working mothers (and here I should qualify this to say that *all* mothers work), i.e., those who work outside the home, must realize that extra effort will be necessary to ensure the well-being of the family.

My husband speaks only French to him and I speak only English.
This is perfectly all right as long as the maid doesn't speak Spanish. As far as I am concerned two languages in the home have no detrimental effect on a normal baby's language development. The use of more than two languages does, however, lead to confusion. So go ahead and by all means give him the benefit of a second language that is so easily and painlessly acquired in this manner.

If I am tense or upset will this affect the baby?
You bet it will. Tension is as contagious as the measles! A baby or child of any age can feel tension and anxiety and will respond in kind. This principle remains true throughout life, although I believe that the infant is even more sensitive to tension than the adult. Much of what is diagnosed as colic is really a reflection of tension in the home.

Any good tips on selecting a baby-sitter?
Observe his or her interaction with your children. Don't entrust your child to someone you have not previously met and seen in action. This means having the sitter over for an orientation session in advance. If you will be away for more than an evening this orientation period is of even greater importance. Plan on a half a day to go over household routines, car pools, and the like. Leave detailed instructions as to what to do in cases of a medical emergency and make sure that your sitter does not have a language problem or else that a friend who can act as an interpreter will be available. Write out a daily schedule for her and list emergency numbers carefully. Make sure that he or she can drive and knows the location of the nearest emergency facility, or will

have transportation to an emergency room if it should become necessary. If away for more than the evening leave a written authorization (prepared with the help of your attorney) authorizing your pediatrician to carry out any medical care he deems necessary during your absence. I would also like to caution against mixing the sexes, particularly with regard to adolescent boys. This can inadvertently lead to sexual exploration, particularly if he is asked to bathe the children and put them to bed.

Are there other suggestions you have regarding sitters?

Be sure that she is old enough to take on the responsibility. For example, to ask a twelve- or thirteen-year-old child to feed two or three children dinner and to wait up until 1 A.M. is just asking too much.

I like to call the sitter from wherever we are in order to make sure that things are going well.

Make sure you tell your children where you will be and approximately what time you will be home and, depending on their ages, make sure that they know what to do in case of an emergency; particularly in case of a fire.

Be fair to the sitter and return when you say you will!

My husband and I want to go on a vacation. How soon can we leave the baby and is there any time that is better than another?

I think that you can plan a trip any time after he is two months of age. As far as optimum time goes, I don't think there is any ideal time as far as your child is concerned. I do not go along with all the so-called critical periods of separation that are frequently talked about. When you feel ready for a break, go ahead and take one.

We are going to fly home to visit the grandparents. Are there any special things I should know about air travel?

In my experience babies behave beautifully on airplanes and no special precautions are needed. They may fly as soon as they reach the ripe old age of two weeks! Occasionally they may have some discomfort with changes of altitude. If he should seem to be fussy, try giving him a bottle. Occasionally the sucking will help to open the Eustachian tubes, those little passages from the nose to the ear that temporarily close with changes in pressure and give you that uncomfortable "blocked up" feeling.

We take the baby everywhere and he seems to be happy and thriving but his grandparents say that we should have a set routine and that what we are doing is harmful. What do you think?

I think that your routine is a bit different from what your parents think it should be. Nevertheless it is your life-style and if the baby seems to be taking to it, I can't see that you are doing him any harm. After all, if this is going to be the family's way of doing things, the sooner he learns to fit in, the better!

What do you think about adoption?

I think it is a wonderful idea. A couple without children is so incomplete, although there are certainly those times when we would all like to be that way!

How should we go about adopting a child?

Contact a reputable agency in your area. Do not try to cut corners and do it "privately." It may prove to be a shortcut to disaster. Sure, it may be a long wait and a lot of the casework may seem unnecessary but in the long run a thorough investigation by a good staff of your desires and needs and the prospective child's is vital in making a successful placement.

At what age should I adopt a child?

Just as early as is feasible, usually under a month of age.

2

Toddlers

Development and Behavior

What are some of the important milestones of development and approximately when should he achieve them?

They include the following:

Rolling over front to back, 3 to 4 months
Rolling over back to front, 4 to 5 months
Sitting alone unsupported, 6 to 8 months
Crawling, 8 to 10 months
Walking, 12 to 16 months

These are, of course, averages and in some cases are a bit later than some sources quote, but in my experience they are correct.

With respect to language development:

Cooing and babbling, 3 to 4 months
Jargon development, 8 to 10 months
Single words, 12 to 24 months

Our daughter is 18 months old. We are planning to visit her grandparents in Chicago for a few days and then fly back East to visit friends in New England before going home. We are then planning to move permanently to New York. Is it all right to travel with her this much or will it do her any permanent psychological harm?

She will probably survive it as well or better than you will. It will disrupt her to some degree and this can be eased by taking along a few familiar and easily transported items such as a favorite stuffed animal. Remember that she will feel some degree of insecurity along the way and it is important to spend some quiet time alone with her since you are the only constants in her environment for a while. Be tolerant of swings in mood, poor eating, etc., during the trip and remember that these are probably the results of anxiety and that all will eventually settle down when you do. There should be no lasting adverse effects from the experience if these general principles are followed.

He wanders about the house at night and I can't keep him in his room even though I've spanked him repeatedly. I just can't prevent it.

Oh, yes, you can. Safety dictates that you must. Having him out of his room and wandering around the house in the middle of the night has frightening prospects. The amount of trouble he can get himself and everyone else into literally staggers the imagination. I am surprised at how frequently this problem is brought to my attention and I must confess that when I first began the practice of pediatrics I had not the slightest idea of how to handle it. Over the years I have developed the following approach. Punish him either with a whack on the behind or whatever other method you feel appropriate. If this is not successful (and all too frequently it is not), then get yourself a chain bolt lock at the local hardware store and use it! The advantage of this device is that he can open the door, see out (and therefore not be frightened) but of course cannot leave the room.

My two-and-a-half-year-old fusses and whines a lot. What can I do?

I recently had an interesting experience in the office. A nice mother brought her two-and-a-half-year-old into the office for his checkup. He began to cry and sob and continued before, during, and after the examination. His mother said that he would do the same thing at home and she was at her wits' end. I then turned to the child and in a firm voice told him to "be quiet" and that I had had enough! He stopped crying immediately and to his mother's amazement was as good as gold thereafter. The point of the story is that we frequently overlook the direct approach, but instead feel too guilty about conveying to the child how he makes us feel. We may discipline him in all sorts of ways—yell at him, bribe him, and so on—but we never really talk to him. I think that the sudden "be quiet" had some impact, but the "I have had enough of your behavior" went across far more effectively. Be honest with yourself and with him and don't be afraid to convey your feelings in a direct and forthright manner.

My two-year-old is not talking as yet. Is this abnormal?

You will want your doctor to advise you on this, but if all other aspects of development seem normal, such as motor development and receptive vocabulary (that is, he seems to understand what is said to him), the chances are excellent that he will begin talking at any moment. Sometimes, instead of developing verbal skills gradually, according to the books, children just seem to talk all at once and frequently talk your ear off thereafter.

My child cries and then suddenly stops breathing when he gets upset. What is the problem?

He probably has breath-holding spells. These usually occur from one to three years of age. First he gets upset (for example, his favorite toy is taken away), then often cries for only a very brief time, then holds his breath causing momentary loss of consciousness and, on rare occasions, even some convulsive movements. He then comes right out of it and seems perfectly fine. Your doctor will want to hear about these spells, but the treatment consists in ignoring them (educated neglect) until he gradually outgrows the tendency. Leaving the room or immediate area as you see him begin to get upset often aborts the attack since these episodes seldom, if ever, occur without an audience. Keeping your cool, once you understand the situation, is very important in the management of breath-holding spells.

He screams when I try to give him medicine. How do I get it down and make it stay down?

Quite a few infants "protest" or, to put it more accurately, scream bloody murder when a teaspoon of anything out of a bottle approaches them. Sometimes using a dropper helps but more often than not this approach meets with the same forceful response. In my experience only the direct and head-on approach is successful in the infant or toddler. This assumes that you have already tried to disguise the evil substance in milk, or even his favorite food, and, contrary to Mary Poppins, a teaspoon of sugar most frequently does not make the medicine go down! Be firm in the beginning and you will avoid even more trouble as he gets older, bigger, and stronger. Hold on and put the spoon in firmly and quickly. If he spits it out or immediately throws it up, repeat the dose right away to show him that you mean business. Usually one or two encounters are sufficient to get over the hurdle. Don't wheedle, bribe, or cajole. This only serves to get everyone worked up and invariably leads to the same unpleasant result. Remember it is a hurdle that he would like to get over as well, for the fear and anxiety produced by a long buildup are just as upsetting to him as to you.

Last summer we were at the beach and my daughter, who was then a year old, loved the water. This summer at age two she seems to be very much afraid. What shall I do?

Forget about it and let her enjoy the beach. She will gradually warm up to it again, but remember, as the child gets a bit older, water often becomes a source of fear until additional experience dictates otherwise. Don't push; respect her desires and don't make a big deal about it.

When should he leave the crib?

This varies a great deal. Some infants begin to climb out of the crib as early as 14 to 16 months of age, but most are content until two years. Those who are early acrobats should make the transition for safety's sake, for once he has learned how to make a fast exit it is too much fun to resist doing it again.

When another member of the family is due to arrive it is important to plan ahead and make the transition from the crib to the bed at least three to four months ahead of time to avoid any feeling of displacement. The older child will need to make enough adjustments, and losing center stage as well as his very own bed may well prove a little too much.

I suggest putting the child in a youth bed (smaller size and lower to the floor) rather than the regular size. It gives a feeling of more security, making for a smoother transition.

What kind of response can I expect from my 20-month-old to the new baby?

Initially, a warm welcome. Sometimes this leads to an excessive amount of handling. He figures that the more love and affection he demonstrates for the baby the better you'll like him. Underneath he usually doesn't feel all that positive about the new arrival; after all, none of us likes to lose center stage. He is also saying that if I'm always around the baby then I'm always where the action is and therefore they can't possibly forget I'm here. You might not think that your 20-month-old is thinking in such a sophisticated manner but you'd better believe it! This stage is often followed by one where he totally ignores the new arrival in the secret hope that he may go away, and, of course, he might want to help things along with a little push now and then, so never leave him alone with the baby. Usually this initial period of adjustment settles down in about two to three months and then there is a rather peaceful interlude when the siblings get to know each other and all is blissful. When the youngest reaches the ripe old age of eight to ten months things begin to come apart again. The oldest feels threatened by the newly acquired motor abilities of his younger sibling, who by now is able to successfully get into his hair at any point. This second major period of adjustment often lasts a bit longer and is frequently more intense than the first, but hang in there. It too shall pass. Nothing is going to eliminate sibling rivalry, which is an important part of normal development. But it will help you to understand it if you look at it from the child's point of view.

My two-year-old has become very "clingy," especially since the new baby arrived. He won't let me out of his sight. How shall I handle it?

It is quite normal for a child to go through this sticky fly-paper stage. He has some concern about being displaced by the baby, which is normal for the age. Be gentle but firm that you are not going to pick him up and carry him around, etc. The more low-keyed and consistent you are, the more secure he will feel about himself and the faster he will work through this stage.

He bites other children. What shall I do?

This is usually a problem around 18 months to two years and can be quickly nipped in the bud by a firm admonition followed by quick removal from the premises. Under no circumstances bite him back or he will begin to think that this is indeed an appropriate way to relate to people.

I think that she is going to be left-handed. Should I try to change her to the right hand?

Absolutely not. Handedness is something that develops early and usually by one year of age it is pretty well established. Not too many years ago left-handed people were stigmatized, but fortunately that is not now the case. Attempts at changing the child to become right-handed result in a great deal of tension, frustration, and anxiety that can only be detrimental. This is true regardless of the age of the child. As to learning ability or success in later life, there is just no correlation to handedness.

What can I do about head banging?

Occasionally I see an infant, most often from ten months to two years of age, who bangs his head forcefully and repetitively against the crib at night. Interestingly, I don't think that this is nearly as frequent a problem as it used to be and I'm not sure why. Anyway, this sort of repetitive rocking motion may also occur without head banging. This type of behavior usually occurs before sleep, either at bedtime or nap time. It is of no consequence and is not indicative of a deep-seated emotional disorder in an otherwise healthy and happy infant. One of my nephews used to bang his head so forcefully that the entire house would shake and he is now doing very well in college. The tendency will gradually pass by age three or four.

What books do you suggest reading regarding my two-year-old child and his general development?

Several excellent books are available which discuss child development in some detail; your pediatrician will be glad to recommend them. I would caution you, however, to try to picture your two-year-old child as he is and not to focus on "the two-year-old child" as he is supposed to be. The appreciation of the individual differences of children is paramount in good child rearing.

Toilet Training

When shall I begin toilet training?

Most children, if left alone, will automatically succeed in learning how and where to deposit their by-products by approximately two and a half to three years of age. The normal child expresses interest in the bathroom at the age of sixteen to twenty months, an interest which should be encouraged. He may want to sit on the pot. Fine, as long as you don't expect him to produce. Let him sit for a few minutes and then pack him up. Don't read him stories, present him with a myriad of his favorite toys, and the like. By the time language is well developed, generally around two or two and a half, he can go into training pants in the daytime. No big deal, just put him in them—you don't need lots of explanation because by now he knows the score. If he balks at the idea or continues to go in his diapers or even elsewhere, then discontinue the whole affair and plan to begin again in another month or two. It is far better to expect him to begin later than to start too early. Keep in mind that they will all be properly "trained" eventually anyway. A few years ago there were advocates of the early approach who began placing the baby on a potty as early at four to five months. There were claims of great success, but what they were developing was a good old conditioned reflex, not a real understanding of what was happening. Current opinion is strongly against this method. Despite all that has been written on the subject, or maybe because of it, there is still perhaps no area of child rearing that produces so many hang-ups. If you are uptight and worried about whether he is ever going to get out of diapers I guarantee that you are headed for trouble. Don't be concerned about whether he will be accepted in preschool next fall either. He'll make it, unless he feels tense and overly anxious, and then watch out because he may not!

My three-year-old was doing beautifully with toilet training but now he is beginning to go in his pants or do his BM behind the door. What shall I do about this unfortunate turn of events?

First of all I would look for any obvious causes of stress and try to alleviate them where practical. Sibling rivalry, too rigorous a school situation, a new baby-sitter or housekeeper are all frequently causes for this regressive behavior. Next I would try not to let it get to me; at least don't let him know that it gets to you. If you do he will suddenly jump to the correct conclusion that he has just acquired an awesome weapon and that all will be wondering as to when and where he will drop the next bomb. It's best to tell him that the toilet is the proper place for such material but once said you do not constantly repeat the same thing nor do you become overwrought. If it occurs again, then quietly, quickly, and with a cool and detached air clean it up as expeditiously as possible, remembering that he will judge the effectiveness of his newly found "weapon" solely on the amount of response he gets from you. As with toilet training in general, keep it in perspective—it is a normal biological function soon to be regulated to the status of habit.

When can I expect him to be fully toilet-trained?

He should be entirely out of diapers and dry at night around his third birthday. If he is not out of diapers in the daytime then you should have a conference with your pediatrician and let him give you some guidelines based on your own individual situation. Don't go on without seeking some practical help. If he is not dry at night, talk it over with your physician, but chances are there is nothing wrong that time will not cure.

I am planning to toilet-train my two-year-old but he is still on the bottle. Should I take this away at the same time?

No, it may prove more than he can handle. I usually start to taper off the bottle around 16 months. It is preferable to have him off the bottle before you put him in training pants.

Do girls toilet-train earlier than boys?

Not only do they accomplish toilet training on the average of six months ahead of boys, but they have far fewer problems with bed-wetting later on. I wish we understood why.

Schooling

When should he start school?

If the present trend continues we will be starting children at one year of age. I have encountered many parents who feel their child will be very much deprived if he is not in a formal, structured school situation by the age of three. To my way of thinking the average child is definitely not ready for any regular school situation until he is at least three years old and in many cases four years. If you watch a group of two-year-olds, for instance, you will note that they play alongside one another without interacting. Besides, he has so many years to go to school; what's the hurry? This is not to say that most children will not benefit by some preschool experience. I think that the public school system is behind the times in not starting formal education at an earlier age than five to six years; three or four years in most cases would seem ideal.

What do you think of play groups and how early can he start in one?

Many people feel that the earlier one starts in a group the better the chance of getting into the college of his choice. Such is certainly not the case and for children under three no play group is necessary. Children of this age do not do much in the way of group play and such a group will not benefit his development. If you're doing it for fun, and perhaps to team up for baby-sitting, fine. A group of a few (three to five) two-year olds, with mothers taking turns watching, is perfectly all right once or twice a week. I do object to highly structured larger groups that meet more frequently.

For more about education see Chapter 16.

GENERAL

The baby fell and bumped his head. He seems fine but I notice a bump on his forehead. Is it serious?

You will want to observe him for the routine signs of head injury, as mentioned elsewhere, but the bump itself is not serious. It is due to bleeding under the skin when he collided with whatever. This "goose egg" will swell in a matter of minutes and then stop enlarging as the pressure of the blood under the skin acts to close off the leak. Thereafter it's a matter of time until the whole thing goes away. Putting ice or cold compresses over the area will often help to reduce the swelling but often it is so upsetting to an already upset child that it hardly seems worth it.

My child seems to have a lot of bulky, loose stools, but he otherwise seems normal. My doctor says he is not concerned.

There are a few children who seem to have a tendency to produce rather bulky and foul-smelling loose stools which can vary in color and sometimes appear green. They may have periods in between where the stools are normal and despite stool cultures and the like no cause is found. This type of child is usually a good eater and grows and develops quite normally until he outgrows this tendency, which may last until he is three to four years of age.

3

Childhood

GENERAL

How do you feel about television?
I don't like it for the most part. One type of child cares little about it while another is a TV addict. He's the guy I'm concerned about. This child will sit transfixed for an indefinite period and needs your supervision. You must ration the amount of time he watches TV very carefully. I think that program quality should be a consideration, but even if the content is excellent, too much of a good thing is still too much. Television can produce an adverse effect on behavior. In fact, if parents complain to me that their child's behavior is really difficult, I will automatically inquire about the TTT (total tube time). If this is on the high side, as it so frequently is, I recommend either reducing TTT dramatically or perhaps discontinuing it altogether. I am beginning to wonder if the photic effect of television (the rapid flickering of light) is not just as important as the program's content in contributing to the so-called TV-addicted child's enjoyment. I strongly suspect that the scintillating photic effect has a lot to do with the pleasurable stimulation some children find with TV. In some cases it is indeed hynotic, and the child sits motionless with a blank expression while watching.

Do you approve of going under the sprinkler in the summertime?
I remember it as being lots of fun and think it's fine as long as the water supply holds out.

Do you approve of children going barefoot in the summertime?
No, I don't. First of all I think you are asking for trouble
with respect to cuts and bruises. I have seen some bad injuries
from youngsters riding their bicycles barefooted. In warmer,
southern climates there are certain parasites such as hookworm
which may gain entry to the body through the soles of the feet.
So keep them in shoes!

Are there any sports activities that you encourage?
Frequent physical activity is as important to the child as it
is to the adult. It is particularly important that your child get
sufficient exercise in the winter months. He should go outside
daily almost without exception. With modern foul-weather gear
inclement days are no longer the problem they once were. Certainly swimming and gymnastics have to head any list of exercises that can be performed year round. Also, they do not
require an opponent or teammates. If he can find an indoor pool,
your child may swim throughout his life.

My child gets carsick. Is there anything I can do to prevent it?
Giving him some antimotion-sickness medication your doctor
suggests about 20 to 30 minutes before going on a trip may help.
Keeping a window down and letting him breathe fresh air and
keeping him occupied with games, conversation, and the like may
also prove helpful but, alas, there is no cure, although in time
most get better.

When should a child learn to swim?
The sooner the better as far as exposure to the water is concerned. There are a couple of basic points to keep in mind: One:
never do anything to a child in the water that you have stated
you will not do. (For example, never push a child off the side of
the pool or let go while he is in the water when you have said
you would not.) Two: don't be goal-directed and insist that
the child must learn to swim at a predetermined age. Instead,
make the experience fun. Frequently a child will learn more
about the principles of swimming by playing in the water than by
attempts at formal instruction. Last: if you don't feel you have the

patience, skill, or understanding, don't try to teach your own children but make sure you provide an opportunity for them to learn from someone else. Most children, with proper instruction, can swim adequately by the time they are five years old. Starting in the middle or more especially the later childhood years is often very difficult and the success rate drops off considerably. So start on it early.

What do you think about organized sports for young children?

I love sports and think that participation is the name of the game. Children in this country are certainly in need of more athletic opportunities. In fact, more recreational facilities for all members of the family are desperately needed. As for organized sports, I have mixed feelings. On the positive side, it is a good experience to be a member of a team, learn the give and take required, and with good coaching and proper equipment, develop skill in a chosen sport. On the negative side is the common philosophy that winning is the only thing that counts, with all the accompanying pressure from coaches and parents. I think we are going through a period where participation has taken a back seat to winning; I hope the pendulum will swing the other way soon.

My 12-year-old daughter seems to have a great deal of body odor. Is there anything I can do about it?

Some body odor is often associated with the onset of pubertal development. A couple of helpful hints: avoid lots of powders and creams, as these frequently will plug up the sweat and sebaceous glands in the skin and accentuate the problem, and tight-fitting synthetic fabrics which don't allow enough air to circulate. Also, keep the skin clean and dry.

His feet smell. What do you suggest?

I sympathize with you; the aroma can indeed knock you over! The almost universal cause is the overuse of tennis shoes or variations thereof. These fit tightly to the foot and therefore do not let enough air circulate to evaporate sweat. Combined with socks made of synthetic fibers they produce an air-tight situation that allows sweat to remain on the skin of the foot. This produces local skin irritation and leads to the multiplication of bacteria and fungi which result in irritation of the skin with peeling, itching, and one awful smell. Treatment consists in keeping the feet clean and dry. To accomplish this, have your budding athlete wear a loose-fitting leather shoe on at least some occasions, wear sandals in warm weather, or go barefoot inside the house. Urge him to change his socks when coming home from school and this will usually cure the problem. No fancy sprays, powders, and the like are usually needed.

What should I tell my child about drugs, and at what age?
He will undoubtedly hear about them and may even be exposed to them in elementary school, probably by the fifth or sixth grade. So, for goodness sakes, don't assume that he doesn't know about them or that he hasn't been exposed to the problem. Your job is to make sure that you touch on the topic at various times in family discussions in an educational way. Make sure that you answer his questions and *listen* to what he has to say so you may judge how much misinformation you must unscramble. The same principles are true regarding cigarettes and alcohol.

My 15-year-old has just started smoking. What can I do about it?
Cigarette smoking among teen-agers is again on the increase. Of course you will want to go over the health facts, and perhaps a session with the doctor might prove helpful. One thing is sure and that is if both parents smoke the chances of the children taking up the habit are quite high. If one parent has the habit they are less, and if neither parent is hooked your child has the best chances of not becoming a victim.

When should I teach him good manners?
From the very beginning. He will learn by observing more than he will by listening. I have a great fear that good manners are becoming a lost art, at least from what I see in the office on a day-to-day basis. Teaching a child that good manners are a way of showing respect for the other fellow is to put the situation in proper perspective. Teaching him to behave in some superficial

automatic fashion is to miss the point. To say thank you and to stand when an older person such as a grandparent enters the room are important in developing a feeling for others.

What do you think about pets and which do you recommend?
I think pets are wonderful. As of this writing we have a dog, hamster, rabbit, and goldfish at home and my six-year-old daughter has her eye on a cat. One should use common sense about acquiring pets. I recently saw a tarantula spider for sale in a pet shop! The age of your child and the amount of care the animal will require need to be considered, and just remember that mother will usually end up doing most of the work. I think it is safest to obtain a pet from a known source such as a reputable pet store or a friend rather than an animal which you know little or nothing about. Your pet should be kept away from stray animals from which you and he may contract diseases. General measures of hygiene and regular veterinary care will prevent any health hazards from developing. Large and potentially very dangerous dogs, such as the German shepherd, seem to be on the increase. You should remember that such a pet is a major responsibility and be particularly cautious with young children around the house. I think the Labrador retriever and Shetland sheepdog are excellent breeds with children.

What is a blood count?
A blood count, or CBC (complete blood count), is a technique that includes the following:

Counting the number of red cells—to check on total production and appearance

Counting the number of white cells to help in diagnosing various kinds of infections ·

Checking to be sure that there are the right numbers and types of white cells

Checking the hemoglobin—hemoglobin carries iron

Checking the number of platelets—these have to do with blood clotting

I noticed some blood in my child's stool the other day. Does this mean he might have cancer?

No, rectal bleeding in children is almost never produced by any malignancy, contrary to adults. Of course, it will need investigation, but chances are it will turn out to be a local cause such as an anal fissure (crack in the mucous membrane or lining of the rectum).

Is cancer a common disease of childhood?

No, I wouldn't say it is common, but it is certainly not rare either. We do see a good deal of it. It is important to stress, however, that the strides in the care of cancer in children have been unbelievable and make the prognosis or outlook vastly more favorable than it was even three or four years ago. The overall picture as to cure and survival is far more favorable than it is in adults.

I notice that my six-year-old has begun to blink her eyes frequently. Do you suppose there is something wrong?

You will want to ask your doctor, but she may well have what we call blephrospasm, frequent eye blinking which is brought on by tension, and which quickly becomes a habit just like nail biting. The treatment for this condition is to ignore it entirely and it will soon go away.

My seven-year-old frequently seems to soil his pants with stool. I have talked to him about it and he says he just can't help it. Can you give me some guidance?

The most frequent cause of this problem is chronic constipation. When the rectum is full of fecal material for long periods of time it becomes dilated or enlarged and this stretching begins to interfere with the sending of signals to the brain as to when a bowel movement is to take place. This results in the leakage of small amounts of stool into the pants at various times during the day. He is just as upset about it as you are, so don't punish him. What you need to do is call on your pediatrician for help. By placing your child on a high-roughage diet and increasing his fluid intake the problem of constipation can usually be easily remedied and the soiling, or paradoxical diarrhea as we call it, will cease.

My child tends to be constipated. What would you suggest I do to help him?

Make sure he gets plenty of roughage and laxative-type foods. Foods in these categories include bran flakes, raisins, prunes, peaches, pears, apricots, and honey, to mention a few.

Make sure he drinks plenty of fluids but watch out for milk as it may be the source of the trouble; you may want to eliminate it from the diet for a while to see if this will help. Water, fruit juices, and the like are helpful.

Make sure that you enlist his cooperation in the effort and explain to him that the goal is to avoid having any discomfort with the bowel process.

Enlist his cooperation in getting him to tell you when he has not gone to the bathroom for over four or five days or if he is beginning to feel uncomfortable. Occasionally enemas will be necessary in order to prevent further discomfort and impaction of the stool.

The goal of all this is to keep the bowel empty a good deal of the time in order to restore normal bowel tone and to ensure proper signals regarding the need for evacuation.

Of course eliminating any punitive attitudes you may have about his constipation and relieving any other areas of tension are also of major importance.

IMMUNIZATIONS

What shots should he get when?

Two months: DPT and polio (oral)

Four months: DPT and polio

Six months: DPT and polio

10 to 12 months: Tuberculin skin test

15 months: Triple vaccine (measles, German measles, and mumps)

18 months: DPT and polio

Four to six years: DPT and polio
14 to 16 years: Td*

D=*diphtheria*
P=*pertussis (whooping cough)*
T=*tetanus*
d=*diphtheria (adult type)*

We are planning a trip to Africa. What immunizations will my child need?

There is an excellent booklet published by the Center for Disease Control and entitled "Health Information for International Travel" (U.S. Department of HEW, Center for Disease Control, Atlanta, Georgia 30333; Publication 76–8280) which should answer your question. The medical service of the U.S. State Department is also a helpful source.

I am just not sure whether he has had all of his shots. What shall I do?

I hear this question all the time. As our society becomes more and more mobile it is increasingly difficult to keep records in order. You should contact your doctor and let him or one of his assistants go over whatever records you have and develop a schedule that will bring the baby up to date. Don't procrastinate about something this important to your child's well-being and don't feel embarrassed; it happens to lots of us. Incompletely immunized children are at greater risk than they need to be, and far too many are in this category. If you anticipate moving and traveling a great deal you should have an immunization record for each of your children in your possession. Such booklets can be obtained from your local health department or your physician's office.

My baby missed his six-month checkup. Will he have to start his immunizations all over again?

No, in all likelihood he won't. There can be a considerable lapse of time between immunizations, but to get the best im-

* Reprinted from the *Infectious Diseases Committee Report of the American Academy of Pediatrics.*

munological response you should try very hard to stick to the schedule outlined by your physician.

What is a booster shot?

This is an injection of a vaccine, or, with polio, a dose by mouth, that is given after the child has received the initial set of immunizations (primary shots). This primary series has resulted in the formation of antibodies which circulate in the body and serve to prevent infection by the specific disease. In time the level of these antibodies begins to drop off but the body still maintains the ability to manufacture them. A booster dose serves to stimulate the body's memory and ability to produce another high level of antibodies, which keeps the immune mechanism in a well-ordered state of readiness.

How important is it that he get all those shots? There seem to be so many. Are they really necessary?

You bet they are. We are so fortunate that most of us have never encountered the diseases against which we immunize, with the exception of rubella (German measles) and mumps. Talk to any pediatrician who was in practice during the days when polio was such a feared disease and you will realize that no well-informed parent would want to risk leaving his child unimmunized. Diphtheria, although rare, is still around and the potential for new cases is constantly with us. It is a potentially fatal disease, as is tetanus, new cases of which are reported in widely distributed areas of the United States each year. Measles (regular measles, rubeola) is a disease that most people think of as rather benign. In truth, measles can cause severe brain damage as well as milder forms of brain involvement. Measles or its complications may even prove fatal. What about the mumps; it really doesn't do any harm other than make you feel sick for a while, does it? Generally, that's so, but occasionally mumps can damage the auditory nerve and lead to deafness. More frequently it can produce an inflammation of the nervous system which may require hospitalization, but from which virtually all children will recover.

Other complications include orchitis, or inflammation of

the testicles, which usually occurs in adolescents and adults and can result in testicular atrophy (loss of the affected testis). German measles (rubella) may have devastating effects on the unborn child if contracted early in pregnancy, producing multiple abnormalities affecting the heart, eyes, and central nervous system, as well as other parts of the body. It is therefore important that children be immunized to prevent the spread of the disease. Pertussis (whooping cough) is another very serious disease that can be fatal or lead to permanent brain damage. It is, like the rest of these illnesses, still around.

All this is not meant to frighten the reader, but rather to motivate you to make sure that your child has received *all* of the recommended immunizations at the proper intervals, including "boosters."

Complacency has led to a situation where the percentage of unimmunized or improperly immunized children is rising at an alarming rate. Not only is it high in the inner-city population where we perhaps need more education programs, but also in the more affluent suburbs. Current estimates run as high as 30 percent in the inner city and 20 percent in the suburbs. All these immunizations can be obtained from your doctor or from a public health clinic, where they are given without charge. There is just no excuse for your child not having them.

LUMPS AND BUMPS

He fell off his bike and scraped his leg. What should I do?

Wash it with soap and water, put on some topical nonprescription antibiotic ointment that contains bacitracin, and cover with some nonsticky gauze pads. It should heal in three to four days. For minor clean scrapes and cuts there is no need for a tetanus booster, providing your child has been properly immunized.

My child cut himself. Does he need a tetanus booster?

The current recommendation of the Committee on Infectious Diseases of the American Academy of Pediatrics is that a child get five tetanus shots altogether for proper immunization: three primary shots and then booster shots at 18 months and four to six years of age. After that a routine tetanus booster is necessary only every ten years. Thus it is not necessary to have your child obtain a booster every time he gets a cut or scratch. Wounds with a high risk of possible tetanus will require a booster and sometimes antibiotics as well (your doctor should decide). This type of wound includes those where there is a great deal of crushed tissue or significant contamination. A clean cut in a properly immunized child, such as one that occurs inside the house, usually does not require a tetanus booster.

My child was accidentally stabbed on the leg with a lead pencil. Will he get lead poisoning?

No, he won't. There is no lead in the lead pencil, only graphite, which will do no harm.

Will a head injury cause fever?

No, usually not. I often get calls about a child who has had a minor head injury followed by vomiting. Of course, the parents are concerned. When I ask about a fever, I frequently learn that the child has a temperature of 102 or so. He is probably coming down with an illness of which vomiting is a part, and the head injury coincidentally occurred at the same time.

EMERGENCIES

He swallowed a penny. What should I do?

An astonishing variety of objects pass through the intestinal tracts of children: buttons, pennies, and marbles to mention a few. If the object is relatively smooth it almost invariably is passed without difficulty and you can check the stool for a few days to be sure. If the object is a sharp one such as a needle, you will want to call the pediatrician. Often nothing special needs to be done; no X-ray is necessary nor must you force fluids or give bread or laxatives. Laxatives may even be dangerous. Each Christmas I'm called about one or two children who have chewed up a Christmas tree ball, swallowing an unknown amount. There has never been any difficulty, not even any bleeding from the mouth. If symptoms of abdominal pain or vomiting develop, you will want to check with your doctor right away.

What should I do if my child chokes on something?

An infant or young child should be held upside down by the feet and pounded firmly on the back to dislodge the object. In the older child turn him head down over your lap or over the side of the bed and again pound on the back. If this fails, pressure applied inward and upward in the upper abdominal area while reaching around from behind the child may be helpful. Let your pediatrician show you how on one of your routine visits. If these maneuvers do not result in clearing the object, reach back with your finger if he is struggling for breath and try to dislodge the foreign body, but be cautious not to push it further back. If the child seems to be exchanging air even though his airway is partially blocked and you have been unable to remove the object easily with your finger, don't force things any further but head for the nearest emergency room.

My child took an overdose of aspirin and my doctor said to make him vomit. How do I go about this?

First give him some lukewarm water to drink and then a tablespoon of syrup of ipecac, which you should always keep on hand. If he doesn't vomit in 15 to 20 minutes repeat the dose, but again try a drink of slightly warm water. Many times this alone will do the job. Syrup of ipecac frequently fails to induce vomiting because no water was given beforehand. If he still does not vomit, then a trip to the nearest emergency room is indicated.

I have heard that certain substances, if ingested, should not be cleared by vomiting.

You are correct. There are two major categories: petroleum distillates like kerosine and corrosives like acid or lye.

What should I do if my child swallows something that might be toxic?

You should have the number of the nearest poison control center and call immediately for advice, if you are unable to reach your pediatrician within a few minutes. Time is of the essence. It is also wise to have syrup of ipecac in the house, but do not use it until you have been advised to do so.

What do the terms first, second, and third degree burns mean?

We no longer use this terminology but instead refer to a burn as either being partial or full thickness.

What is the most common cause of burns in children?

Scalding with hot water is the most frequent type of burn. Boiling water that is knocked off the stove causes a very serious type of burn that is usually what we call full thickness: it destroys the skin. Burns caused by hot coffee, tea, etc., usually result in partial thickness, as the hot water has in fact cooled slightly after being poured into the cup.

What should I do if my child burns himself?

Whatever damage to the tissue that has been done was done the instant the burn occurred. You can certainly make him more comfortable if, for example, it is a small burn of the finger, by applying ice, which relieves pain and may also help to reduce some of the swelling. Covering the burn with grease or Vaseline is also helpful. This applies to minor burns, which are characterized by small areas of redness. A burn which blisters, covers a wide area, seems quite deep, or is in what we call a critical area (the face, palm of the hand, sole of the foot, genitalia, or nipple) should be seen by a physician. If the burn is fairly extensive, of course, you will want to get him to a medical facility promptly. To cover a burned area use plastic kitchen wrap, which will keep it clean and also will not stick to the surface while you transport him to the doctor.

How should I handle a burn that blisters?

I think that any burn that blisters should be seen by a physician. If the blisters are intact it is wise to leave them alone since they contain rich body fluid that protects the burned area from infection and promotes healing. If the blisters are broken, the dead skin should be removed. Full-thickness burns do not blister, which means that blistered skin has suffered a less serious injury, leading to a better long-term result.

Should a burn be treated by the open or closed method?

I am asked this question quite frequently. Essentially it is something your doctor should decide but, generally speaking, while severe burns which require hospitalization are often treated by the "open" method, most of those we see are in the minor category and will need some sort of local dressing. This is to prevent any infection from occurring in the burned area, something which can cause additional skin damage and result in more scarring. It is simply not practical to keep an active child clean without applying some sort of bandage. Great strides have been made recently in combatting infection and there are several excellent new local antibiotic creams as well as newer nonadhesive dressings that make the treatment of burns far better than was the case several years ago.

My child got his finger caught in the car door and I think the end is just about off. What should I do?

Obviously you should rush him to the emergency room but it is important to remember that if the finger should indeed be severed, you should bring along the dismembered part, as the success rate of reimplanting it is very high.

What about a cut on the face?

Here we are very much concerned about the long-term cosmetic effect and because of this, even though the laceration (cut) may be relatively insignificant, it should be sutured with great care. If it is large, a plastic surgeon, if available, is often called.

I know that it is important to treat facial cuts properly, but what about one in the eyebrow?

This is just as important since if it does not heal properly it may lead to irregular growth of the eyebrow and be even more of a cosmetic problem than if it were elsewhere on the face. Such a cut should be properly closed with stitches.

My child fell and cut his tongue. Will he need stitches?

Most small cuts inside the mouth, including the tongue, do not need any stitches and will heal by themselves quite rapidly. They seldom become infected because the inside of the mouth is normally so full of bacteria that the tissue there is quite resistant to infection. Larger cuts or those which by their location may cause trouble (for example, those involving the gums) are exceptions to the rule.

My child just cut himself. Will he need stitches?

If the wound is through the outer layer of skin and the skin edges are separated (pulled apart), chances are he will. If it is a small cut and not too deep you may try a butterfly bandage (or better still, some of the newer tension strips available at the drugstore), which you should have on hand in the medicine cabinet.

How soon should the sutures be put in?

Within a few hours, if possible, in order to prevent infection from developing. If a delay of several hours is unavoidable, wash the area well with water and soap, put on some local antibiotic ointment, and cover with a sterile, no-stick gauze pad.

He has just had stitches put in. What shall I do to take care of them and when should they be removed?

Keep the sutured area clean and dry, covered with the sterile dressing that was put on at the time. It is a good idea to change the dressing in 48 hours. Check if there is any redness and swelling extending out from the sutured area, a sign of infection. If it is a large dressing, your doctor may need to change it, but if it is small you can do it yourself. I think it a good idea to put a small amount of a local antibiotic ointment over the area, such as bacitracin which you can buy without a presecription. Be careful not to touch the area with dirty hands.

As a rule sutures which are placed in the face can be removed in five days. If left in longer they may produce further scarring. Those in the arm or leg can usually be taken out in seven days and the same is true for those in the scalp. Sutures placed over movable areas of skin, such as the knee, for example, may need to stay in 10 to 14 days and if removed too soon the cut may reopen when tension is placed on the skin as it moves over the joint area. Although you could probably remove some sutures yourself, I feel that it is a good idea to have your doctor or some trained medical person do it. At times it can be more difficult than it appears and occasionally only a portion of the sutures may be removed at a time if healing is not complete.

What is a butterfly bandage?

This is a most useful bandage and should be in the family medicine closet. You can either buy them already made up or in a pinch you can make your own out of a standard Band-Aid. Essentially the design, resembling the wings of a butterfly, enables you to put tension on either side of a cut, thus holding the skin edges together. Many small cuts can be closed in this manner, avoiding the traumatic experience of having it sutured (stitched). It should be left in place for approximately one week's time. Recently, various tension strips have become available which can effectively close many small cuts.

What is epiglottitis?

It is one of the few real emergency situations that arise in pediatrics and you should be aware of its symptoms. It is an illness which is caused by a bacterium (Hemophilus influenza) and which starts *abruptly* with some cough, *hoarseness*, and difficulty in *breathing*. The child may soon begin to drool and gasp for breath. Unlike croup, which occurs predominantly in the one to three-year age group, this condition is usually found in the older child (six to ten), although it may occur at any age. The inflammation and swelling of the epiglottis, which is a normally small piece of tissue down behind the tongue, can progress rapidly and lead to blockage of the airway. If your child shows any of these symptoms you should call your physician immediately and if he is not available head for the hospital.

What should I do if I have a real emergency?

If there is a good local rescue squad, call them. If not, take him to the nearest hospital emergency room. Do not wait to try to call the doctor. Just go and go quickly. Know where the nearest hospital is located beforehand. Remember, do not waste time trying to locate your doctor by phone. Even if he is there he may not be able to reach you in time. When you arrive at the emergency room you can have the people there contact your physician. If in doubt as to whether it is an emergency, play it safe by assuming it is.

We are in the process of restoring a very old house in the city. Right now it is a mess as we are having all the paint removed, replastering, etc. I have heard that there might be some danger from lead. Is it true?

Yes. Older houses frequently contain lead-based paint and dangerous levels of lead can accumulate in the air under such conditions. If you have any doubts check with your pediatrician; he may want to have a blood-lead level done on the family members.

What should I have on hand in the medicine cabinet?

Aspirin.

Syrup of ipecac—to induce vomiting after accidental ingestions.

Auralgan ear drops—for that earache that invariably begins in the middle of the night when all the drugstores are closed.

Sterile gauze—the nonstick type.

Antibiotic ointment—one containing bacitracin is best.

Band-Aids—particularly the butterfly or tension strip variety, which can be used to close small cuts, avoiding the necessity for stitches.

Ice bag—can be used for sprains and bruises and also as a hot-water bottle, very helpful for an earache.

Vaporizer—I like the cold-steam kind best since most of the time the child is already warm with fever.

Phone numbers of pediatrician, emergency rescue/ambulance service, police and fire departments, poison control center.

Thermometer.

Nasal syringe.

GROWTH

When will my daughter stop growing?

Approximately two years after the start of her first menstrual period.

Is it true that girls are generally ahead of boys in development?

Yes, it is. For example, studies have shown that with regard to bone maturity girls are approximately one month ahead of boys at birth.

He is so small, doctor. What can be done about it?

First of all have your physician plot his height and weight on a growth chart. He may well not be as short as you think.

There are only two situations in which short stature may need further investigation. One is where the child's growth rate has slowed down; where, for example, he was in the ninetieth percentile for height at age three, and at age four is in the tenth percentile. The other is where both parents are very tall and the child is quite small, let's say below the third percentile. Short stature is one of the most frequent reasons why children are referred to the endocrinologist, but seldom is any hormone deficiency or other abnormality found. Only in very rare instances is there need for any therapy with growth hormone.

Can you tell me something about growth rate for children?

Immediately after birth there is some weight loss, which is then quickly regained. This is followed by a dramatic rate of growth which up to four months of age proceeds at the rate of just over one inch and approximately one and a half pounds per month. After the fourth month growth slows down and by two years of age the boy has reached approximately half his adult height, the girl having done so at eighteen months. Throughout the childhood years the growth rate proceeds at approximately two and a half inches per year until adolescence, at which time there is another dramatic growth spurt.

She is so tall. What can we do about her height?

By giving hormones one can accelerate sexual maturation and therefore bring bone growth to a halt. It is, however, very difficult to prove that this will actually result in a shorter person than would have been the case without hormone therapy. In addition there are many possible short- and long-term adverse side effects of such therapy and therefore no treatment is usually recommended. I see many tall girls in the office, but I see just as many tall boys, and I figure that they will have plenty of company.

What about growth hormone?

Growth hormone does just what its name implies. In very rare instances an individual is deficient in this hormone and will respond to treatment with it. If no deficiency exists the hormone will have no effect. This hormone is not easily obtained since it must be extracted from human pituitary glands; it is only given in very special situations.

What about growing pains? Are there such things?

Yes, they certainly do exist. The cause is unknown although most people think they have something to do with rapid growth and perhaps some degree of muscle imbalance. They are most frequent in the five to seven-year-old. The child may awaken at night complaining of pain in the legs, which is frequently relieved by gentle rubbing. Almost always the pain is in both legs or varies from side to side. If the pain is localized in one leg it should be evaluated further. These pains seem to be more frequent after vigorous exercise and the child appears healthy in all other respects.

SEXUAL DEVELOPMENT

My four-year-old wants to know what his penis is called. Do you approve of other names or should I use the adult term?

Tell it like it is. Don't use made-up names for parts of the anatomy. This will only produce confusion for your child and give him the idea that there is something improper about sexuality in general.

When do you think I should teach my child about sex?

I believe he should learn as he goes along and not on a periodic formal lecture basis. He will begin to ask questions at an early age and you should answer them in a straightforward and honest manner. He will observe sexual behavior in pets and perhaps even in the home by accident. He will be exposed to some sexual education beginning in the early school years, if not in the classroom, then by his peers on the playground. Make sure you have an ongoing dialogue and don't save it all up for the famous birds and bees lecture because chances are that by this time he will either know the answers or have so many misconceptions that it may be too late to orient him in the right direction.

He masturbates. What shall I do?

All children masturbate and there is no reason for concern unless it becomes excessive. Make it clear that it is not acceptable behavior in public, then ignore the whole thing. Often children masturbate at times when they are bored or have nothing else to do, and you should divert them while avoiding a direct confrontation. Keep in mind that it is a universal, normal phenomenon and that it occurs in both sexes.

My little girl has a vaginal discharge.

A vaginal discharge is frequently seen in little girls and is usually of a thin, whitish consistency. It is most often self-limited but if it persists check with your doctor. I have found that wearing loose-fitting cotton underpants is a great help in clearing vaginal irritation since the synthetic materials and particularly tights or pantyhose fail to let enough air circulate to the genital area. This produces increased warmth and moisture, which sets the stage for bacteria to proliferate and produces a vaginal inflammation and subsequent discharge. The use of bubble-bath soaps can also produce skin irritation and even a more generalized skin eruption. Having her sit in a tub of plain warm water twice a day as well as aerating the area as much as possible will clear most vaginal discharges. A thick yellowish-green or persistent discharge should be checked by your doctor at the outset since it may indicate infection or even the presence of a foreign body that has been inserted in the vagina.

Is there any way I can predict how soon my child will develop sexually?

Generally, the short, stocky child will develop before the tall, slender one.

Should my child see me naked?

Be natural, remembering that privacy and modesty are indeed natural instincts. It is not desirable to go traipsing around nude in front of the children, as this can produce psychological problems, since the adult body is considerably different from the child's. Likewise, modesty carried to extremes gives the child the idea that there is something terribly wrong with seeing the body uncovered.

At what age is my daughter likely to start her menstrual periods?

The following are general averages: white girls, 10–16 years; black girls, 9–14; Oriental girls, 11–16.

My daughter's periods are so irregular. She hasn't had one in three months now. Is this unusual?

Because of immaturity of the hormonal system (like any other piece of machinery it needs time to warm up and run well), she is likely to have a considerable amount of irregularity of menstrual periods for up to three to four years after their onset.

There is a small nodule under my child's nipple. What shall I do about it and what is it anyway?

We frequently see a small "nubbin" of tissue under the nipple as the first sign of breast development in the girl; it usually begins on one side rather than symmetrically. You'll just have to face the fact that she is indeed growing up. This phenomenon usually takes place around nine to ten years of age.

What if I notice the same thing, but it's a boy?

Pubertal boys, ages 13 to 14 on the average, often show some breast enlargement with nodularity under the nipple area. This is usually tender to the touch, as it is in girls. There is one major difference, of course: it goes away in the boy.

My 14-year-old son has recently developed some enlargement of his breasts. Is this abnormal?

Chances are it is perfectly normal gynecomastia, frequently seen in pubertal boys. It is interesting that the more masculine or virilized boys seem to have a higher incidence of breast enlargement. This is because they have more androgens (male hormones), from which estrogens (female hormones) are produced. In time the enlargement spontaneously subsides, and no treatment is necessary.

Is it all right if my daughter starts out using tampons instead of pads during her periods?

Yes, it is perfectly all right.

NUTRITION

What are some so-called junk foods?

Many of those foods that contain "empty" calories—that is, foods that contribute only calories, fat, and carbohydrates. Often, these are the things to nibble on that come in plastic bags, cereals with all kinds of sugar added, various snack foods, and soft drinks. All such foods should be sharply curtailed in your child's diet.

Will eating a lot of sugar produce diabetes?

No, it will not, but it certainly is not a good idea.

My child is very much overweight. I'm sure there must be something wrong with his thyroid gland.

It is important to remember that well over 95 percent of children who are obese are also tall, and since thyroid deficiency produces small stature this gland, although much maligned, is seldom at fault. Like it or not, the problem is that he just takes in more calories than are needed.

My child is overweight. What can I do?

We try to keep a tight rein on excessive weight gain starting with the first-month visit. Teaching good nutrition to parents, and later to their children, is basic to good pediatrics. Let's face it, some of us have a genetic predisposition to excessive weight gain which is not fully understood at present. I try to spot these children early and suggest to the parents, while they still have control over the diet, the avoidance of excessive caloric intake. We used to believe that the faster the baby gained the healthier he was and the better we were as parents. This idea has radically changed, of course, and an excessive or improperly balanced caloric intake has become more of a problem in our country than undernutrition.

Frequently a sibling is as thin as a rail and perhaps one, or occasionally both, parents have never had a weight problem. I urge these parents to make proper nutrition a family affair (as it should be anyway) and to discuss principles of proper eating at mealtime and as a family unit. Avoid singling out the child with a weight problem and emphasize that all members of the family must consider good nutrition, not just overweight and underweight. A child may not be overweight at all, but be malnourished because of improper diet. Considering the matter in this healthier and more realistic perspective avoids increasing the anxiety level in the youngster who is overweight, an anxiety which frequently leads to more compulsive eating. There is just nothing worse than the rest of the family "suffering" without their favorite dessert because one child has a "weight problem." One often hears, "I don't keep anything like that in the house because he will eat it all." It should be, "I don't keep any of it in the house because I don't think it is nutritious."

Also helpful in the management of the obese child is a visit to the doctor for a weight check at five to six years of age or even younger if the child and family appear sufficiently well motivated. The child can relate to the doctor as a more objective outsider and, for this reason, I usually have the parents, particularly of the older child, wait in the reception room while I talk with the child alone. Even though no weight loss may be apparent for a while, as the child grows in height the relative weight loss becomes more apparent. The visits should be scheduled every three or four weeks at first and the goals set low enough that the child can feel successful—losing one to two pounds in a month, for example. During this time the physician is showing a positive interest in the child's problem and not placing all the responsibility on the parents. However, if one parent is overweight and exhibits poor dietary habits, it is going to be even harder for the children. If both parents are in this category it will be almost impossible!

I do not prescribe a specific diet for the overweight child, but only a general reduction in the quantity of food, particularly carbohydrates. You should try to get across that, yes, you can eat ice cream, or a piece of cake; just don't overdo it. Each individual has a different metabolic situation and the child can be taught to recognize or even feel when he has gained too much and cut back accordingly. You're dealing with a lifetime situation; keep this in mind.

Are there any special diets you recommend for children who are overweight?

No, I don't recommend any of the many "fad" diets for children. There must be a new one publicized every month but none is proved to be either effective or safe for children. Furthermore, you are trying to teach the child how to eat properly for the rest of his life, not simply to lose weight in a hurry. The fad or crash diet has absolutely no place in dealing with children.

My child is so thin. I just can't seem to make him eat. What can I do?

I'm sure you have had him checked out by your doctor, but if you haven't, you should. The chances are overwhelming that he will pass his examination with flying colors and you will be told that there is nothing wrong with him. Accept this advice. Many children have slender body builds and many appear downright scrawny, yet are among the most active children with the most endurance. Body build is an inherited characteristic and probably others, somewhere in the family, are just like him. He is always going to be thin and when he is an adult everyone will consider this the healthy way to be! If you try to push food in to "fatten him up," you may later be trying your darnedest to keep his weight under control instead.

My child seems tired and listless and has a picky appetite. How about a tonic?

I am frequently asked this question. I know of no general tonic which will correct your child's problem. Certainly you will want to confer with your pediatrician and if he finds a specific deficit such as iron deficiency (checked by a hemoglobin test), he may want to prescribe iron. Or, if there are signs of a vitamin deficiency—a rarity—he will treat accordingly. Do not just go to the drugstore and buy some sort of "tonic."

What about all the additives and preservatives in food? Do you think they should be avoided?

As a general rule, yes. Although the scientific evidence against various additives and preservatives is often meager or nonexistent, we're all beginning to believe that more natural and unadulterated food is better for you. We are certainly on the threshold of a nutritional revolution in medicine where we will significantly improve health through the findings of the nutritional sciences.

Are vitamin deficiencies common in children?

No, not in our country. The overwhelming majority receive more than enough vitamins.

The following are frequently and *mistakenly* attributed to vitamin deficiency:

> He is tired all the time.
> He has dry skin.
> He frequently catches colds.
> He has a picky appetite.
> He is small.
> He is so thin.

What about megavitamins? Are they good to give to my child?

No, it is not a good idea. The American Academy of Pediatrics Committee on Nutrition recommends that no supplemental vitamins are necessary over and above the daily requirements, which are set by the Food and Drug Administration. Since so many of the foods that the child eats are fortified he does not need any further vitamin supplementation if he eats a reasonably balanced diet. Remember that excessive amounts of vitamins can be toxic and the long-term administration of abnormally high levels may produce as yet unknown undesirable side effects.

4

Infection

FEVER AND ASPIRIN

What are some good indicators of how sick the child might be?

Lethargy—Most sick children are listless to some degree, but if the child is really lethargic, particularly even after sponging or taking aspirin, and if this lethargy seems constant (he does not have periods where he perks up and seems much improved), then this is a danger sign.

Vomiting—This frequently occurs with childhood illness, but persistent vomiting is a danger signal.

Loss of appetite—This is an excellent indicator of the degree of illness. The more severe the loss, the more severe the illness.

Poor color—Marked pallor or, on rare occasions, even blueness means a serious problem.

Fever—A temperature that persists at high levels and is not amenable to sponging or aspirin.

Diarrhea—Frequent, explosive, and watery stools are a serious matter, as loss of fluid through the gastrointestinal tract can produce rapid dehydration, particularly in the small infant.

"He doesn't look right"—A very important observation in the infant.

"He doesn't act right."

Persistent crying—If he continues to cry despite all attempts to comfort him by picking him up, changing the diapers, etc., then there is something wrong that needs investigation.

Difficult breathing.

Generalized or localized jerking movements that may indicate a convulsion.

Decreased urination—Means depleting of body fluid.

Stiff neck in association with fever and/or generally not feeling well.

What are the most common illnesses you see in the office?

Upper respiratory infections, otitis media (middle ear infections), and gastroenteritis (vomiting and/or diarrhea).

Are there different ways to take the temperature?

Yes, there are three basic methods.

Oral (by mouth)—should not be attempted in the young or uncooperative child since he may bite down on the thermometer. The thermometer should be kept in the mouth a full three minutes to be accurate and therefore taking oral temperature is difficult in most children under eight years of age.

Axillary (under the arm)—an inaccurrate and difficult method since the thermometer must be kept in place a full five minutes, which is no easy matter with a sick child.

Rectal—the best method and certainly the most accurate. Three minutes are required for an accurate reading.

Feeling with your hand is a totally inaccurate method of gauging temperature. The normal body temperature is from 97° to 100.5° Fahrenheit, and is usually higher in the late afternoon and evening than in the morning.

Because so many of my patients come from countries outside the United States and are used to taking the temperature in Celsius, and because our country is also gradually adopting the metric system, I thought it would be helpful to include a conversion table of Celsius to Fahrenheit.

$$98.6° \text{ F} = 37° \text{ C}$$
$$100.4° \text{ F} = 38° \text{ C}$$
$$102.2° \text{ F} = 39° \text{ C}$$
$$104.0° \text{ F} = 40° \text{ C}$$

Is the degree of temperature proportionate to the severity of the illness?

No, frequently it is not. Fever is the body's response to infection and is a sign that the body is in combat against the invader. The degree of fever depends on the type of infection, its location in the body, and the individual's thermostat. Many infants and children will consistently run very high temperatures with relatively minor infections. But a child can be very sick with only a slight elevation in temperature. In small babies a few days of age, subnormal temperatures can be a sign of serious illness. All in all it is far better to base the decision on how the child acts in general, rather than on the degree of temperature.

Two good general rules regarding fever are:

1. If your child has a temperature of 24 hours' duration you will want to check in, even if he has no associated symptoms.

2. *Any* infant under three months of age who develops a fever can have a potentially serious infection even though he manifests no other symptoms.

If his temperature goes too high is he likely to have a febrile convulsion?

This is one of the reasons we like to control the temperature and, by use of aspirin and sponging, keep it from rising too rapidly to high levels such as 104 and 105. Some children are going to have febrile convulsions and there is no way to know in advance which ones will. Usually they occur with the initial rise in fever and early in the illness. They are usually of very short duration, less than a minute, and do not cause any brain damage.

Does the fact that he has had a febrile convulsion mean that he will have epilepsy?

No, it certainly does not. The overwhelming majority of children who have a seizure with fever either never have another one or outgrow the tendency entirely and are perfectly normal children in every respect.

Will high fever cause brain damage?

Fever is a normal response of the body to infection and signals that the child is actively combatting the infection. It is exceedingly rare for fever itself to do any damage to a child since it almost never reaches levels high enough to produce any brain damage. Temperatures of 103 to 105 are seen frequently in pediatric practice.

Do certain children tend to run high fevers?

Yes, some children develop temperatures of 103 and 104 with relatively minor infections. These children are usually in the one- to four-year-old age group. It is as though their thermostats are set a bit higher.

What is the proper aspirin dosage?

One grain (one children's aspirin tablet), which is actually one and a quarter grains but close enough, per year of age up to age five where one can use four children's aspirin tablets or one adult tablet, which is equivalent in dosage (five grains). Aspirin may be given every four to six hours, but remember we must look for the cause of the fever. Only give aspirin if he has fever or feels uncomfortable.

There has been so much publicity about the dangers of aspirin poisoning that it has become widespread to give far less aspirin than needed, in my experience. The following is a good dosage schedule:

4–8 months: ½ grain (½ children's tablet)
8 months–1½ years: 1 grain (1 tablet)
1½–3 years of age: 2 grains (2 tablets)
3–5 years: 3 grains (3 tablets)
5–10 years: 5 grains (4 tablets or 1 adult tablet)
Greater than ten years: 5–10 grains (1 to 2 adult tablets)

Suppose he is vomiting with the fever. Is there any other way to give aspirin other than by mouth?

You will certainly want to talk to your pediatrician if the child has fever and is vomiting. To answer the question, yes, aspirin is available in suppository form and can therefore be given rectally if necessary.

Do you prefer aspirin or nonaspirin compounds?

Unless there is a specific aspirin sensitivity I prefer aspirin.

How do I sponge the baby and when should I do so?

This is a technique with which all parents should be familiar. I usually recommend that it be used if the temperature is *over 104* rectally. Mix one part of rubbing alcohol with two parts of room-temperature water. Soak a towel and wrap the infant with this, changing it frequently and rubbing gently to increase circulation to the skin. Usually 30 to 40 minutes is enough. Remember it is easier to sponge early before the temperature has reached a high level for a considerable length of time. The purpose of the alcohol is to increase the rate of evaporation of moisture from the skin as it is through the process of radiation that heat is lost from the body. Cold water should not be used, not only because it causes further discomfort, but also because it may induce shivering, which counteracts your efforts by increasing body heat from the muscular activity generated.

MANAGING THE SICK CHILD

What is meant by incubation period?

This term is used to denote the time from the entrance of the infective agent into the body until symptoms of the disease appear. It may vary from one day to several months. The individual is usually not contagious during this period and thus need not be isolated from others.

Should I wake him in the middle of the night to take his temperature?

This is usually not necessary; if his temperature goes up very high he will wake up of his own accord. Usually the temperature drops after midnight and is at its lowest in the early morning hours and at its highest in the evening.

What are some good foods to give my child when he is sick?

Remember that all children will lose their appetite when sick. "Light foods" are best: soups, broth, toast, crackers, Jell-O, yogurt, boiled chicken, soft-boiled egg, ginger ale, Coca-Cola, and tea with sugar are all in this category.

Should I wake him in the middle of the night to give him medicine?

Many medications are to be given every six hours or four times a day, but usually it is not necessary to wake the child in the middle of the night. It is more important that he get a good night's sleep, and the same is true for you. Your doctor will probably tell you specifically if he wants you to wake him up.

Is it necessary to give many antibiotic shots to children with infections?

No, fortunately it is not. In office practice we seldom need to give any medication by injection since the oral preparations are very well and quickly absorbed and achieve as good a blood level as they do if given by "shot." Occasionally if the child is vomiting or in the case of some streptococcal infections an injection may be necessary.

Is there any special time to give antibiotic medicine?

About an hour or so before meals is the best time since the medication is absorbed more effectively through an otherwise empty stomach.

Which is better, the cold or the warm mist vaporizer?

Not everyone agrees on this one, but I prefer the cold mist vaporizer. For one thing it is safer since occasional bad burns have been caused by the hot-water type. Secondly, it has a cooling effect in the room and the child who needs it frequently has a fever.

What should I put in the vaporizer?

Just plain water. No other special preparations are necessary.

What does a vaporizer do, anyway?

It helps to liquefy mucus in the respiratory tract and that makes it more easily coughed up.

Can vaporizers themselves cause a problem?

Yes, they occasionally can. There are some children whose condition seems to be aggravated by their use. Also molds may proliferate in the vaporizer and in an allergic child add insult to injury, so make sure that the unit is kept clean.

If I have some medicine left over, will it keep? I hate to throw it away, especially since it was so expensive.

Your doctor usually will prescribe just enough medicine for the illness he is treating. This is particularly true with anti-biotics, and therefore you should not end up with anything left over. If you do, toss it out since an antibiotic in liquid form will soon lose its potency and will just be a safety hazard. One of the commonest errors is to stop the medication as soon as the child is feeling better, which results in the strong possibility that the infection will soon produce symptoms again since it has not been fully eradicated. Decongestants, cough medicines, and the like may be kept on hand depending on how often your child has a particular medicine prescribed, but don't load up the medicine cabinet as you are only inviting trouble.

I have several bottles of medicine but I have forgotten which is which.

You would be surprised how often this situation occurs. Don't ever accept a prescription from the druggist that is not clearly *labeled* as to its contents and how it is to be taken.

My pediatrician mentioned that he was going to check my child's antibody levels because he gets so many infections. Could you tell me what he means?

There are several techniques for determining the amounts of various antibodies which circulate in the blood and this procedure has even been adopted for office use. The best known fraction of the total antibody is the gamma globulin but there are several others of importance. Occasional children who have repeated infections may indeed lack enough antibody or even produce none at all. If the difficulty is in the gamma globulin fraction, then injections of this substance on a periodic basis may prove helpful in controlling the incidence of infection.

Suppose he has something contagious like chicken pox. Won't he expose other children if I take him to my doctor's office?

Not if you call ahead and set up a time so that on your arrival he can be quickly placed in an examining room, preferably one set aside as an isolation area. Don't take him unannounced!

Is it safe to take him out to the doctor's office if he acts very sick or has a high fever?

It is perfectly safe to take him into the office and his acting sick is all the more reason he should be seen, preferably in the office or hospital out-patient facility, where various tests can be performed.

If he is sick should he stay in bed?

Not necessarily. The best rule is to play it the way he feels. Most infections do not require that he stay in bed.

Can he go outside if he is sick?

If he has a minor illness such as a cold, moderate temperature elevation (101 to 102), and above all, if he doesn't act very sick, then going outside for a bit of fresh air on a nice day is certainly not going to harm him.

There seems to be a lot of illness in our community this summer. Do you think that the swimming pool is a factor?

There is very often a good deal of illness in the summer and I can't blame it all on the neighborhood pool. That is not to say that the pool is not the source of a good deal of infection, for it certainly is, and for two reasons. First of all many viruses can be spread through the water, and second there is a good deal of crowding which increases the chance of infection not only in the pool but in the locker room as well.

He has a normal temperature now and the doctor says he is all clear of infection but he still is tired and has a poor appetite. What can I do?

Wait a few more days and he will gradually bounce back. The infection took something out of his system and it takes time for him to get back in full swing. This convalescent period is quite normal.

When can he go back to school?

For the most part, after his temperature has been normal for 24 hours, providing he otherwise feels up to it.

We are going on a trip to Europe. What do you suggest we take with us in the way of medication for the children?

As a general rule I do not like to give out a lot of medications to take along since I am always concerned that the wrong one may be given at the wrong time and it seems to me that it puts more responsibility on the parents than they should rightfully assume. I think some mild antidiarrhea preparation is about all that is generally needed.

UPPER RESPIRATORY INFECTIONS

What is meant by the term URI?

It stands for upper respiratory infection, and is used more or less synonymously with common cold. Another term occasionally used is *acute coryza.*

When my child goes to the doctor for a respiratory infection he does a throat culture. Why?

A throat culture is a simple office procedure that can provide your pediatrician with valuable information. Studies vary as to its accuracy, but all agree that it is more accurate than relying on clinical judgment alone. But, like any laboratory test it can be inaccurate and *does not* replace the doctor's judgment and he may wish to treat your child with antibiotics before getting the results or even if the culture is negative. Most frequently your doctor is determining whether your child has strep throat. If he does, he will need antibiotic treatment. Penicillin is the drug of choice unless for some reason he is unable to take it. Your doctor will also look for other types of bacteria but they will not necessarily be treated with antibiotics. He is mainly concerned about the strep since, if untreated, it can (in rare circumstances) cause complications involving the heart, kidneys or joints.

What is strep throat?
The term refers to a throat or tonsil infection caused by a bacteria known as the streptococcus.

He was just diagnosed as having a strep throat. When is it safe to let him play with other children?
As a general rule, most children with streptococcal infections of the throat are no longer contagious after 48 hours on the appropriate antibiotic. He should be recultured after he completes the treatment to make sure it has been eradicated. In addition, cultures of those with whom he has been in close contact are also indicated.

Is it true that some children are more prone to streptococcal infections than others?
Yes, it is, and certain families have a high recurrence rate of streptococcal infections for reasons we don't fully understand.

What is scarlet fever?
Scarlet fever is an illness produced by the streptococcus that causes a sore throat, fever, and a red rash; another name is *scarlatina*. Strep throat is virtually the same illness except that there is no rash present. It responds dramatically to antibiotic treatment, with penicillin being the medication of choice.

My doctor said the throat culture was negative. What does this mean?

Check with your doctor, but chances are he means that no streptococcus was found on the culture. Your child may still need an antibiotic, however, and if he is not improving you should check back with your doctor. Most often upper respiratory infections with no involvement of the middle ear clear up without the use of any antibiotic. The increased use of the throat culture has definitely decreased the use of antibiotics—a good thing.

COLDS

Should I give my child extra doses of vitamin C? I have heard that it will prevent his getting colds.

I wish we did have such a simple remedy to prevent the common cold but, alas, it looks as though we don't. Recent studies tend to show that giving vitamin C seems to make no difference whatsoever with regard to the frequency or severity of colds although there is still some difference of opinion over this matter. Just because a certain amount of something works in the body doesn't mean that more of the same will do even more for you. This principle is true no matter what you are considering.

He seems to get so many colds. What can I do?

Very little. Chances are he is in the peak age group, which is from two and a half to five years of age (although occasionally an immune deficiency or underlying allergy plays a role). During this very susceptible period you will really get to know your pediatrician well, if you don't already. Take heart; by the time he is six or seven you will probably only see him once a year for the regular checkup!

Will chills and dampness cause a cold?

Despite the lack of objective scientific evidence on this point I believe that cold wet weather predisposes the individual to the development of colds. No one is a greater advocate of the outdoors than I am, but make sure that your child is dressed appropriately before going out. The foul-weather gear now available for all ages makes it possible to get outside for a family outing in almost any weather.

Is it more important for a parent deliberately to keep a child away from other children who have colds or should you expose him, in moderation, in order to develop immunity?

I don't think it is a good idea to deliberately expose a child to any illness.

I have heard that there may be some new cold vaccines on the way. Is this true?

Although work is being done in this area no successful vaccine has yet been developed.

STOMACH INFECTIONS—VOMITING AND DIARRHEA

What does the term stomach virus *refer to?*

Usually this term is used in place of gastroenteritis. It is a condition most often caused by a virus but occasionally by bacteria; vomiting and diarrhea are usually present to varying degrees along with some fever.

What causes diarrhea?

For the most part, infectious diarrhea in children is a self-limited illness caused by viruses. Recent evidence suggests that a specific group of viruses known as rheoviruses may be the cause of a great deal of diarrhea in the pediatric population.

My two-year-old has diarrhea. What can I give him to eat?

If the diarrhea is fairly pronounced, that is, if he is having loose, watery bowel movements, then the idea is to rest the bowel by giving foods that produce a minimum of digestive activity. I like to start with a liquid diet which includes:

Sugar water (one-half teaspoon of sugar to four ounces of water).

Ginger ale—Give it "flat," that is to say, after the dissolved carbon dioxide has bubbled off.

Coca-Cola—Flat; avoid colas without sugar as they can lead to low blood sugar if given in great quantity and to the exclusion of sugar-containing drinks.

Weak to medium-strength tea with sugar.

Avoid juices of all kinds, particularly apple.

Avoid milk. As the diarrhea improves, skimmed milk may be used but do not boil the milk as it can produce dangerously high levels of sodium.

As the diarrhea improves one may add broth; rice cereal; toast, crackers; banana, raw apple, or applesauce; cottage cheese; yogurt; soft-boiled egg; Jell-O (avoid exotic flavors).

This dietary regimen will take care of most cases of diarrhea. The most frequent error is not knowing what to give and trying to return to a normal diet too quickly. In my experience, so-called antidiarrheal medications are seldom needed.

Loss of fluid by the body, in this case through the gastrointestinal tract, can produce dehydration, which is the most frequent serious complication of diarrhea and the one that most often requires hospitalization. Therefore it is important to keep giving the child fluid. You should check with your doctor. If there is a good deal of vomiting present, which is often the case at the very beginning of gastroenteritis, then resting the stomach by giving nothing at all for two to three hours may prove helpful. Following this period fluids may be started by giving small amounts, i.e., two to three ounces at a time, and then waiting 15 to 20 minutes before repeating the same amount. If one attempts to give too much at a time, nausea and vomiting frequently ensue.

What are some signs of dehydration that I should watch for?
They include the following:

Decrease or absence of tearing.

Dryness of the mouth caused by a reduction in the amount of saliva.

Decrease in both the frequency and the amount of urination.

Listlessness.

Decrease in the elasticity of the skin. When you pick up a fold of skin on the tummy, it should snap back immediately.

A doughy feel to the skin.

What should I give my two-year-old who has been vomiting?

Your doctor will usually prescribe a "light diet" once the vomiting is brought under control. This includes weak tea with sugar, ginger ale, and sugar colas after they have been allowed to go "flat" (lose their carbonation) since this can produce gas in the tummy and only worsen the situation. Juices usually aggravate the situation, as does milk. Plain water is usually nauseating, something few people seem to know. The byword is small amounts at frequent intervals, and no solid foods until he is really keeping the fluids down for 12 to 24 hours or so.

What if he is vomiting as well as having diarrhea?

You will want to check with your pediatrician, but if he advises dietary treatment use the same liquids as recommended for diarrhea. The trick here is to give small amounts at frequent intervals. For example, two to three ounces should be followed 10 or 15 minutes later by another two to three ounces. Frequently the child may be thirsty and want to take a large amount in one gulp, but this usually serves to distend an already upset tummy and produces further vomiting. If a sudden wave of vomiting begins, as it often does when the gastroenteritis or "tummy bug" hits, then it is best to give nothing for an hour or two until it passes and then begin with fluids. With regard to both vomiting and diarrhea we must watch for signs of dehydration, the body losing more fluid via the vomitus and/or stools than is taken in. This can lead to dangerous consequences and you should be familiar with some of the signs of dehydration, as listed above.

My child had a stomachache last night. The doctor said he had gastroenteritis, but how would I know if he had appendicitis?

The most important sign of appendicitis is pain, which usually comes on gradually and becomes steadily worse and is constant and unrelenting. Fever, nausea and vomiting, loss of appetite, and constipation are frequently associated. At times this can be a very difficult diagnosis to make and therefore it is a good policy to check with your doctor if your child has persistent pain—certainly if it lasts more than an hour—if it is recurrent, or seems unusually severe.

EAR INFECTIONS

Why are ear infections so common in children?

There are probably several reasons. First, the Eustachian tube, the canal that leads from the nose to the middle ear, is shorter and straighter in the child; as he gets older, it angles upward, making it more difficult for bacteria to enter the middle ear. Second, certain immune mechanisms which fight bacteria are not as well developed in the young child. Third, the youngster has not had sufficient exposure and time to develop antibodies against many of the bacteria that cause ear infections, and lastly, underlying allergy may play a role. There are undoubtedly more factors that are poorly understood at present.

What is meant by the term ear infection?

There are two types of ear infections: swimmer's ear, which refers to inflammation of the external ear canal, and middle-ear infection. The latter is usually associated with a cold and causes painful inflammation of the eardrum. Most ear infections develop as secondary complications on top of a cold or allergy and the majority are caused by bacteria. The mode of infection is from the nose through the Eustachian tube into the middle ear. These infections occur on the inside of the eardrum and are not due to cold air or bacteria entering from the external ear canal. The usual therapy involves antibiotics and some form of decongestant to help open the Eustachian tube and nasal passages and aid in draining away the infection.

Can he have an ear infection without any fever?

Yes, many children have repeated ear infections with no associated elevation of temperature, while others almost always run some fever. It is important to recognize your child's own pattern of response to illness.

He seems to get ear infections. Is there anything I can keep on hand when he cries in pain in the middle of the night?

Yes, several forms of drops are available that will relieve the pain and, believe me, there is nothing more painful or miserable than an earache. Ask your doctor to prescribe some for you to keep on hand. If you happen to be stuck somewhere and don't have anything to give while waiting to see the doctor, a couple of drops of warm olive oil will help, as well as a dose of a decongestant that your doctor recommends.

What do you think about the value of decongestants and antihistamines in preventing middle-ear infections?

I think if properly prescribed by your doctor they can be of great help not only in preventing ear infections but also in making the child more comfortable during one.

Are ear infections contagious?

The ear infection per se is not contagious but the virus or, in most cases, the bacteria that causes the infection can be transmitted to another person. It may then produce or not produce an infection and may or may not lead to an ear infection in that person.

What is swimmer's ear?

Swimmer's ear (external otitis) is an infection of the skin of the ear canal that is most frequently caused by bacteria, but occasionally by a fungus. It is usually aggravated by excessive water in the ears from swimming. In this condition bacteria enter from outside into the ear canal, whereas in middle-ear infections they enter through the nose and mouth through the Eustachian tube and locate in the eardrum.

What can be done to prevent swimmer's ear?

The best method of prevention is to use plain rubbing alcohol in the ears. Insert several drops in each ear after swimming. This not only helps kill bacteria but also aids in evaporation of moisture in the ear canal.

His ear hurts. Is there some way of telling if it is swimmer's ear?

Yes, frequently you can tell the difference. Pull on the earlobe or wiggle the ear. If it's swimmer's ear he'll give a holler because by performing this little maneuver you are moving the canal itself. If he has a middle-ear infection chances are it will not affect him one way or the other.

Will covering the ears prevent ear infections?

Middle-ear infections are caused by infection which spreads from the nose through the Eustachian tubes that connect to the ears. They do not result from infection entering the external canal and covering the ears in winter will therefore do nothing to prevent them.

My child has had several ear infections this winter and I am wondering if he will build up resistance to the antibiotics which he has taken.

No, the body does not build up immunity against the antibiotic but bacteria that cause infection can. This happens with occasional long-term administration of an antibiotic in large doses for a serious infection. Also, the more a particular antibiotic is used throughout the population the more likely the bacteria for which it is intended are to develop resistance. For example, there was a time when virtually all staphylococci were highly susceptible to penicillin and could be eradicated with ease. Nowadays most staphylococci are resistant to penicillin. Getting back to your question, it is perfectly all right for him to take the antibiotics as prescribed by your doctor. Each is given for a specific infection and for a short period of time. What we all tend to forget is all the dreadful complications from infections which occurred before the advent of antibiotic therapy. I do not condone the unnecessary administration of antibiotics, but neither do I worry much about complications from the treatment as long as it is given appropriately.

What is a ruptured eardrum?

The most common cause of a ruptured or perforated eardrum in children is a middle-ear infection, so-called otitis media. Because of the inflammation in the middle ear pressure builds up behind the eardrum. Unless the condition is treated (and in some cases even when it is) the pressure may cause the eardrum to rupture. Pus will then be able to drain out of the ear canal. This is nature's way of decompressing and draining the ear and, of course, in the preantibiotic days it was a frequent occurrence. Either the eardrum perforated spontaneously or a small hole was cut in it in order to drain the ear. Nowadays we do not see many perforations, but those we do are usually very small holes which heal within 24 to 48 hours and no permanent damage has been done.

CHICKEN POX AND MUMPS

What does chicken pox look like?

The child usually has symptoms of a mild cold and then breaks out with small pink spots fairly widely scattered beginning on the trunk, but also on the scalp, face, and literally everywhere. Some of these spots will have a small blister in the center filled with a clear liquid, others will just be pink, and some will have already had the blistered area (vesicle) scratched open. The rash literally breaks out while you are watching, is itchy, and is in various stages of eruption.

How long is he contagious with chicken pox and what is the incubation period?

He is contagious from 24 to 48 hours prior to the development of the rash until one week after he breaks out. The incubation period (time from exposure to coming down with the illness) is two to three weeks. Incidentally, he is *not* contagious during the incubation period and therefore need not be isolated.

Is there any way to prevent chicken pox?

No. We know that it is caused by a virus, but most attempts to grow it in tissue culture have failed and we as yet don't have any vaccine to prevent it, at least in this country. Recently a vaccine has been developed in Japan that sounds quite promising.

He has the chicken pox and his grandparents are planning to visit. I have heard that there can be some danger to exposing older people. Is this right?

Yes, you are correct. Elderly or chronically ill individuals can develop herpes zoster (shingles), a very painful skin condition from exposure to chicken pox, even if they had the disease when they were children. These two conditions are caused by the same virus.

Is it true he can get the mumps even though he's had the mumps vaccine?

Yes. Although the vaccines for German measles, mumps, and measles have an excellent record, there are still occasional breakdowns, particularly with the mumps vaccine and more recently with the measles vaccine as well.

He has the mumps. When can he go back to school?

When the swelling has gone down, usually about one week from the onset.

He has some swelling near the jaw. Is it mumps?

If the swelling is *up over* the jawbone and in front of the ear, if it is diffuse (that is, you cannot tell its exact borders), and if this area is tender, then it's probably the mumps.

TICKS, WORMS, AND LICE

How do you remove a tick?

Take a piece of gauze, or, better still, tweezers, making sure to grasp the tick firmly, including the head, and pull. Don't use your bare hands. Wash up carefully. In areas where there are a lot of ticks it is a good idea to check the children twice a day, looking particularly in the scalp where they love to hide.

My doctor says my child has pinworms. What are they and how did he get them?

These are small, round, whitish, threadlike worms which are frequently found in children as well as their parents. They require a human host, so don't blame your pet. The problem is that the eggs, which are laid in the perianal area, rub off on sheets, towels, fingernails, and the like and may remain viable for months. The best way to break the cycle of infection is to treat all infected family members and to make sure that the children's fingernails are cut short and that they wash their hands regularly. Your doctor will prescribe the appropriate medicine. Symptoms of pinworms are rectal itching or occasionally vaginal itching. There seems to be some difference of opinion among physicians as to whether they cause other symptoms such as abdominal pain, but in my experience they can. Pinworms may be diagnosed by looking for the adult worms around the anal area first thing in the morning or by doing a simple Scotch tape test of the perianal skin and looking for the eggs under the microscope. Their presence, although surprising, is no cause for panic or great alarm; they are extremely common and easily treated.

What is ringworm?

This is a skin infection caused by a fungus and not by a worm. Your doctor will prescribe some medication which should clear it up. Don't worry; it is not all that contagious.

Can my child catch ringworm from the dog or cat?

He certainly can, and if he has a case it would be wise to take a good look at the skin of the family pet.

My child has been scratching his scalp a great deal lately. Could he have lice?

Yes, he may well be the victim of head lice. In recent years there has been a virtual epidemic of head lice across the country for reasons that are not fully understood, especially since it used to be considered a medical curiosity, found only in the poorest of living conditions. The situation has now radically changed and lice are in all areas of our society. If you suspect them, look closely through the scalp for a brownish transparent insect. Also look along the hair shafts for the egg casings, or "nits."

What is the treatment for lice?

A special shampoo is very effective. Consult your doctor since it requires a prescription and should not be used without medical advice.

How did my child get lice in the first place and what should be done to prevent their recurrence?

Lice are spread from person to person. They live only on humans and therefore your dog or cat is innocent. The eggs may lodge on the bedclothes. They can be in hairbrushes or combs, and these should be cleaned and boiled thoroughly. To prevent cross infection in schools, where transmission usually takes place, it is necessary to inspect the children for head lice periodically and exclude those with active infection until they have been properly treated.

I haven't seen any lice and I have used the shampoo as my doctor directed, but I can still see little eggs in the scalp. Does that mean that he is still infected?

No, it does not. Since your child has been properly treated, the eggs have been killed, but they may remain on the hair shafts for quite some time. They are in fact very difficult to remove fully, but they will not hatch and can do no harm.

ANIMAL BITES—RABIES

What are the animals that are most likely to carry rabies?

Dogs, cats, skunks, foxes, raccoons, and bats are the most frequent carriers of the disease.

My child was bitten by a dog. What should I do?

Wash the area well with soap and water and put on a sterile dressing. I like to use a topical antibiotic ointment as well, and I think it a good idea to have one on hand. As a general rule the dog should be observed for ten days to make sure that it is healthy. With a pet this, of course, can be done by the owner. If it is an unknown dog make sure it is picked up by the police and does not wander away since, if not found, the child may need to be treated for rabies. With any animal bite it is of the utmost importance to keep tabs on the animal so that it can be observed for any signs of illness. You will want to check with your doctor regarding the need for a tetanus booster.

My child was bitten by his pet hamster. Is there a danger of rabies?

Bites of rabbits, squirrels, hamsters, guinea pigs, gerbils, chipmunks, rats, mice, and other rodents almost never result in human rabies in this country and therefore do not usually call for antirabies prophylaxis.

OTHER INFECTIONS

I've noticed some lumps in his neck. What are they?

They are small nodules of lymphatic tissue called lymph nodes which are scattered all over the body. They are soft, small (less than pea-sized), and movable. Many are found in the tissue just under the skin. When the body is fighting an infection these glands or nodes enlarge, as they are busy producing antibodies to stave off the invading bacteria or virus. They especially enlarge in the area of infection if it is localized in one part of the body. For example, if there is an infection of the scalp, the lymph nodes along the back of the neck will enlarge. If there is an infected area on the leg, the glands in the groin on that side may enlarge. With upper respiratory infections the glands in the neck, which are connected to the throat area, will noticeably increase in size. Usually they will remain enlarged about a week or two. Of course, if one should continue to enlarge or become tender or inflamed, the doctor should see it. All lymphatic tissue is more prominent in children, so that one can frequently feel small pea-sized nodes in various places. This is particularly true in the child under seven or eight years of age.

He has swollen glands. What does this mean?

This term is used to describe the enlargement of lymph nodes which occurs in children, particularly those in the younger age groups, in response to infection. They are frequently enlarged in the neck but can be felt many other places as well. They subside as the infection clears.

What is a stye?

Is is an infected gland among the margin of the eyelid. Usually, warm compresses and some local antibiotic eye ointment will clear it up promptly.

Are sinus infections common in young children?

No, they're not. Most of the sinus cavities are not well developed until the child is six or seven years old, and therefore sinus infections become more frequent as he gets older. Sinus headache is usually not a problem in the young child and other causes for headache should be ruled out before one applies this diagnosis.

What is croup?

Croup is a sudden swelling of the vocal cords that is most frequently caused by a viral infection. It comes on very suddenly, with only minor associated cold symptoms, usually beginning in the late afternoon or night. It occurs most frequently from one to three years of age. There is immediate difficulty breathing air *in*. The narrowed passage results in noisy breathing, a barky cough just like a seal's. You will want to check with your doctor and he can frequently judge the severity by listening to the child breathe over the phone. If there is associated blueness and severe restlessness (fighting for breath), this is an emergency situation. Most of the time the child will respond to steaming in the bathroom and the use of the vaporizer (a cold steam is best). This should be used in conjunction with a tent that can be made with sheets over the crib or bed so as to concentrate the mist. Propping him up with several pillows also will make breathing a great deal easier. Most of the time steaming, use of the vaporizer, and calmly holding him will take care of the situation. If he is able to take fluids and to sleep it is a sign that the attack is relatively mild, although he make wake several times during the night. Antibiotics are usually not indicated for this type of infection, but your doctor will want to order some type of cough medicine.

Usually croup lasts three nights, each with a milder attack. Each morning the child may feel fine, show no evidence of any difficulty, and be bouncing around, but by late afternoon or evening will start to have difficulty again. One last tip—if he fails to respond to the vaporizer and steam, taking him out briefly and well wrapped into the cold night air frequently has a beneficial effect. This undoubtedly explains why many children rapidly improve during the trip from the house to the emergency room of the nearest hospital.

What about the recent measles outbreak in various parts of the country? Is it necessary for my child to be reimmunized against measles?

Children who received measles vaccine before one year of age should be reimmunized. In addition, in the face of a measles outbreak infants at risk of exposure may be immunized as early as six months of age. In order to ensure permanent immunity the vaccine should then be repeated at 15 months of age.

What is mono?

The term *mono* refers to infectious mononucleosis, a disease caused by a virus. It can occur in young children, although more often it infects adolescents and young adults. The illness produces fatigue, sore throat, low-grade fever, and general malaise. There is no specific treatment and the child most always recovers uneventfully.

What is "walking pneumonia"?

This term is left over from the old days when the patient was able to walk around but suddenly became very ill with an overwhelming infection. Fortunately, this is a term of the past and most pneumonia we see is viral in origin, not serious, and clears without complications.

Is pneumonitis different from pneumonia?

No, it's not; the two terms are used interchangeably.

What is Christmas tree disease?

This is a wonderful name, far preferable to the medical term. It is a self-limited viral illness that produces a fine, bumpy rash which is particularly prominent over the trunk and more especially the back. Its distribution follows a Christmas tree pattern (diagonal) and hence the name. Frequently a single large patch signals the beginning of the disease. At times the rash may be mildly itchy, but no restrictions on activity are necessary. We think that the disease is caused by a virus, although none has been isolated. Sunlight helps. The rash may last from two to six weeks.

What is a Tine test?

This is a skin test used to determine if the child has been exposed to tuberculosis sometime in the past (positive test). If it is positive it does not necessarily mean that he will become ill with tuberculosis, but it does mean that at some point the bacillus has entered the body. It is very important that he receive this skin test periodically (most pediatricians do it once a year) in order that we may be sure at what point it has become positive. At present it is recommended that INH, an antituberculosis drug, be given children for one year after a positive TB skin test has been confirmed, since they are more susceptible to developing symptomatic tuberculosis.

Can a virus be cultured, and if so, why doesn't my doctor culture my child for viruses?

Viral culture requires a good deal of sophisticated laboratory equipment. The virus requires living tissue on which to grow and may take weeks before enough is grown for any positive identification. To date viral culture techniques are beyond the capability of the physician's office and because of the long time interval required are of little practical help in the management of acute illnesses.

Are canker sores caused by a vitamin deficiency?
No, they are not. They are caused by a virus.

I recently heard that smallpox vaccination was no longer being routinely given. Is this true?
It certainly is. The U.S. Public Health Service no longer recommends routine smallpox vaccination in the United States. A case of smallpox has not been seen in this country for many years and the possible complications, including death, from smallpox vaccination are felt to far outweigh any risk of contracting the disease. The only exceptions are medical personnel and those traveling to areas of the world where they may still encounter the disease.

There is a case of hepatitis in my child's school. Should he have a shot to prevent it?
Not if he has had no direct close exposure. Gamma globulin is recommended for all household contacts as well as other close contacts of patients with hepatitis. For the most part the disease is spread through the oral intestinal passway.

What about the risk of hepatitis in other parts of the world? We are planning a trip to Spain.
I think it is worthwhile to give gamma globulin injections in the hope of preventing hepatitis if you are traveling abroad. This is particularly important in areas of poor hygiene and in those along the seacoast where contaminated water may be a source of hepatitis. If at all in doubt, I would tend to get the injection.

What is roseola?
This is a viral infection which produces a very high fever, 103 to 105, for as long as three to four days. Following the resolution of the fever a fine reddish generalized rash appears and quickly fades within 24 hours. The rash occurs after the temperature returns to normal. This infection occurs most frequently in the six-month to two-year-old group. Despite the high temperature the infant does not usually act very sick and often is up and

playing around. It is a very low-grade contagion and no specific treatment is indicated.

What is Rocky Mountain spotted fever?

This is an illness produced by a rickettsia, an organism sort of halfway between a bacteria and a virus, and carried by the dog or wood tick. The incubation period is from one to eight days and the disease is characterized by fever, headache, nausea, vomiting, muscle aches, and usually a fine reddish rash that begins on the arms, legs, hands and feet, and spreads inward. Proper antibiotic treatment usually results in a prompt cure. If you live in an area infested with ticks, you should make it a habit to check the children as well as yourself twice a day in order to remove any ticks from the body. (Pay careful attention to the scalp.) Since it requires several hours for the tick to become attached and begin to feed, this is the best method of prevention, along with wearing clothing that covers the body when in a heavily infested area, and making sure that your dog is kept as free of ticks as possible and is not allowed to roam through the woods at will.

What is impetigo?

Impetigo is a bacterial infection of the skin. It usually occurs when there is some (often unseen) break in the surface of the skin through which bacteria enter. Often these areas occur around the nose and mouth and frequently have a wet, oozy appearance. You should check with your doctor as to what treatment he recommends.

What is molluscum?

Molluscum contagiosum is a commonly seen skin infection of children that is caused by a virus. It causes little pink raised bumps on the skin and is treated by opening them in the office, a simple and painless procedure.

What is Fifth disease?

This frequently encountered illness usually begins with a diffuse redness of both cheeks. This is followed in a day or two, sometimes sooner, by a fine, lacy, flat, reddish rash that is particularly pronounced over the outside surfaces of the arms and legs. There may be a low fever, but most often the child feels fine. This is another pediatric illness that we think is caused by a virus but as yet none has been isolated. There is no treatment and no need to isolate the child. The course is variable, but the rash may last for several weeks, often coming and going before disappearing altogether.

For more about skin and its infections see Chapter 11.

5

Urinary System

URINALYSIS

Is it a good idea for my child to have a urinalysis done?

Yes, it is important that a urinalysis be performed. Ideally the first urinalysis should be done under a year of age. Because the urinalysis can be normal and the infant can still have a urinary infection, it is probably a good idea to have a urine culture done on the specimen as well. Thereafter a urinalysis should be done periodically by your doctor. We are finding more and more urinary infections at a younger age as we begin to search more for them. This type of infection can produce many different symptoms such as "colic," diarrhea, and unexplained fever, to mention three. It can be the underlying cause of poor weight gain and general failure to thrive. Like many things in medicine, the more diligently we search for a condition the more frequently we seem to find it.

What does a urinalysis check for?

Specific gravity—The ability of the kidney to filter and concentrate the urine properly.

Protein—If present, an indication of possible kidney disease.

Sugar—If present, an indication of diabetes.

Acetone—If present, an indication of possible dehydration or possibly of diabetes.

Blood cells—Normally a few white blood cells are present, but if there are many or if red cells are present, then a disease of the urinary tract or blood is also likely to be present.

In addition to a routine urinalysis done as part of the child's yearly examination it is also important that he receive a urine culture sometime in the first two years of life and again at school age since the presence of urinary infection cannot always be excluded by means of a routine urinalysis.

CIRCUMCISION

What if my baby is not circumcised? Is there anything I need to do?

Make sure that you fully retract (pull back) the foreskin to reveal as much of the glans as possible. This should be done once daily. With the passage of time you will find that the entire glans will be exposed, but this may take up to one or two years. Ask your physician to show you how to retract the skin.

What if the infant has hypospadias, but we are orthodox Jews and would like to have a ritual circumcision?

Don't worry. A ritual circumcision can be performed in which blood is let, but no skin is actually removed.

What is hypospadias?

This is a condition where the opening of the urethra is not located at the end of the penis. In the mildest and most common form the opening is in the head of the penis but just under where it should be. This type is not serious at all and requires no correction, as there is no impairment of function. Other types of hypospadius may require extensive surgical treatment. A circumcision should not be done until the infant has been evaluated by a physician, as the foreskin may be needed for surgical repair of the difficulty. There is an increased incidence of other genitourinary abnormalities with hypospadius, so your physician will want to evaluate him carefully.

Is there any special care to be given the circumcision?

It is a good idea to make sure that the skin is fully retracted over the glans at least once a day. This applies if there is any skin left down over the glans itself.

INFECTIONS AND IRRITATIONS

Is it true that urinary-tract infections are common in children?
Yes, indeed. Approximately 5 percent of all girls will develop a urinary infection and a great number also occur in boys, although they are not as frequent. One reason may be that in girls the urethra is a very short tube, which makes it easier for bacteria to enter the bladder, but there are no doubt other factors which we do not fully understand.

Are urinary-tract infections contagious?
No, they're not.

What are the symptoms of a urinary infection?
Increased frequency of urination; discomfort associated with the passage of urine; occasionally, but not usually, fever.

How can I prevent my daughter from getting a urinary infection?
There is no way to prevent urinary infections other than using good local hygiene, and even this is no sure bet. Remember that babies constantly stool in the diaper and this fecal material inevitably gets around the urethral area. Yet the vast majority do not develop urinary infections. This indicates that proper wiping, so emphasized by parents and many physicians, while certainly a good idea, probably has little or no effect on the incidence of urinary infections. Rather, it seems that various immune mechanisms are at work which are poorly understood at present.

How about about bubble baths and various other soaps? Will they lead to urinary infections?
These substances, especially bubble baths, will produce considerable skin and urethral irritation (local discomfort), but they do not contribute to the development of a urinary infection.

Will sitting on a cold floor cause a urinary infection?
No, it will just give you a cold bottom.

Will drinking a lot of cranberry juice tend to protect my child from developing urinary infections?

I wish it would but I know of no evidence that says it will.

How about going around in wet pants or wet bathing suits? Will this cause a urinary infection?

The answer is no. It will, however, produce local skin irritation.

What about irritation of the genitalia in little girls?

It is certainly not uncommon and can be produced by inflamed skin or mucous membranes caused by various soaps, bubble baths, and the like. This type of irritation can produce discomfort on urination just like a urinary infection. A urinalysis and urine culture are indicated to differentiate the two conditions. Another frequent cause is the wearing of tights and underwear made of synthetic fabrics. This type of clothing frequently produces an airtight situation that allows moisture to accumulate and irritate the skin. Loose-fitting cotton underpants, although not so stylish, are a great help in clearing up local irritation.

What would you suggest regarding treatment of this kind of local irritation?

The best treatment is the sitz bath, which consists of sitting in a tub of warm water a couple of times a day. Do not use any detergent or perfumed soap. For the first day or so just plain water is enough; then you can use a bland, nonirritating soap and rinse off well. You may have been told that tub bathing can cause urinary infections in girls but this is not true; therefore there is no need to encourage her to take showers.

What is a bladder infection?

This is an infection of the urinary bladder (cystitis), most often caused by bacteria. The symptoms are frequency of urination along with a sense of urgency and discomfort. There may occasionally be some blood in the urine as well and there is usually no fever or at best a low-grade one, 101 for example. Frequently the child becomes incontinent of urine—that is, he loses all voluntary control. Treatment consists of sitz baths for local comfort and appropriate antibiotic treatment, preferably after a urinalysis and urine culture have been done.

How serious is a kidney infection?

This is more serious than a bladder infection. It is relatively uncommon in children. All the symptoms of a bladder infection are present, but in addition there is usually fever that can run very high, shaking chills, and the child appears acutely ill. This condition requires immediate treatment and your doctor should be consulted right away.

Is back pain frequently a symptom of kidney disease?

Contrary to what you may have heard, back pain is rarely a symptom of any renal (kidney) problem. A kidney problem will usually elicit numerous other complaints, such as discomfort and frequency of urination, fever, chills, and the like.

WETTING

My child wets in the daytime. Is this serious?

In children over five years daytime wetting should be considered abnormal; the most common cause is a urinary-tract infection. The condition should be evaluated. In younger children, the cause may also be infection, but most frequently it is because of immaturity.

He wets his bed at night. How shall I handle it?

Bed-wetting, or enuresis, is a very prevalent problem. It is six times more common in boys than in girls, for reasons we do not understand. I can remember being a counselor in a boys' camp and being presented with a typewritten list of all the bed wetters and their cabin numbers so that they could be awakened each night. So take heart, yours is not an isolated problem. No one as yet has come up with an acceptable explanation as to the causes of enuresis, although there are a myriad of different ideas on the subject. I do not believe it is a psychological problem. I have seen far too many otherwise perfectly well-adjusted children who are bed wetters. Most of the time children who are bed wetters are deep sleepers who are just about impossible to wake up, so there seems to be more of a physiological type rather than a psychological one. Usually there is no problem in the daytime, and there is no reason to go poking and prodding. Your doctor may want to do a simple urinalysis and urine culture to rule out the possibility of a urinary infection. This is a simple procedure and can be done right in the office. Instrumentation and X-ray procedures are not necessary unless the problem continues past age six or seven and then your doctor may feel differently. Gradually a child will learn bladder control at night but it may take him several years to do so.

Do you have any practical suggestions for management of enuresis?

Yes indeed. First let me point out that in my experience restriction of fluids has absolutely no effect, and that I am also against the use of drugs in the treatment of enuresis. Not only do the latter have occasional bad side effects but more importantly if they work at all the patient usually relapses after stopping the medication and nothing has been accomplished. Sometimes waking the child just before you turn in for the night is helpful but all too frequently it is also a failure. Punitive measures such as making him wash out the sheets are to be condemned; he usually feels bad enough about it anyway. I do feel that discussing the situation with the child is a positive way to handle things. Giving him the idea that he can influence the situation is worthwhile. Keeping a calendar and awarding a gold star for dry nights or using a point system—ten points for each dry night, five lost for wetting, a prize or special treat when he achieves 100 points— can be helpful. If for no other reason they show the child that when he exerts a strong positive desire to stay dry he can frequently be successful. Very frequently a child who is enuretic will not have an "accident" if he stays at his grandparents' house or sleeps over with a friend. Thus, although the problem is not one of emotional maladjustment in my book, still it is not a totally involuntary process. Giving him the idea that he can and should participate in correcting it reverses the feeling of helpless passivity that many children develop concerning bed-wetting. Removal of any obvious causes of overfatigue or stress and making sure there is plenty of positive emotional support on the home front are also important.

Do you advise any special medications for enuresis?

No, I do not. Furthermore, I am not an advocate of the bell system, in which urination activates a bell by breaking an electrical circuit. In the older child, wetting may produce a great deal of emotional trauma and various attempts at counseling of parents and child may have failed. Only in these exceptional instances drug treatment, and even the use of a bell device, may be indicated. By far the most successful form of treatment is to understand that this is a universal problem, that it is a normal variation of development, and that the child himself, with the help of time, a relaxed attitude, and strong positive support, can voluntarily influence the situation.

How long is he likely to be a bed wetter?

Prepare yourself! It can persist until age 10 or 12 and occasionally even later. Most children (approximately 80 percent) are dry at night by four years of age. Most of those who continue beyond this point usually dry out by six to seven years.

MISCELLANEOUS

My four-year-old is constantly going to the bathroom. I read somewhere that the reason is he has a small bladder. Is this true?

No, there is no such a thing as a small bladder. His pressure gauge is just set for a smaller volume and he therefore never allows the bladder to fill fully. Often there is some anxiety present that only adds fuel to the fire. As he gets older he will outgrow the so-called immature bladder. This condition needs no treatment other than time.

He seems to go to the bathroom a lot in the daytime yet he stays dry at night. Is there anything wrong?

Frequency of urination in the daytime only is far more common in boys than girls and is usually the result of anxiety. It reaches its peak at about four to five years of age. In the absence of discomfort or other evidence of illness, and with a normal urine examination, reassurance usually handles the problem. Many times the amount voided at any one time is quite small, and frequently he drinks excessive amounts of water during the day as well. Downplaying the whole thing is the most effective treatment.

My son got his penis caught in his zipper. What should I do?

Take a pair of scissors and carefullly cut out the zipper from the pants. Put on his bathrobe and take him to the doctor.

I have noticed that when my little boy urinates, the urine goes off to one side.

Deflection of the urinary stream is caused by a small piece of tissue inside the urethral meatus. This acts very much like putting your finger in front of a hose; it does not obstruct the flow but merely changes its direction. Unless he constantly hits the wall or his brother's shoe, it needs no correction and he will learn to compensate as he aims. In severe cases it is easily corrected by a simple surgical procedure, but this is rarely necessary.

My little girl fell on her hobbyhorse and I notice that her genital area is quite bruised. Is this serious?

A straddle injury, as this type of trauma is called, seldom produces any harm in girls. A small mucosal laceration may sometimes cause some minor bleeding and perhaps some swelling and discoloration that will disappear in time. In boys this type of injury can be quite serious, as it can damage the urethra.

I noticed some blood in the urine. What shall I do?

Blood in the urine is always abnormal and requires evaluation by the doctor. Blood in the urine following injury is a medical emergency and the child should be seen by a physician immediately.

Sometimes I have noticed that my little boy's testicles are not in the scrotum. Where do they go, and is this OK?

In boys we often see what is known as a retractile testicle. This is one which can easily slide up the inguinal canal (groin area). This frequently occurs in response to cold but can happen for no apparent reason. The testicle later slides back down into the scrotum. This condition may occur with one or both testicles and is perfectly normal and needs no treatment.

His testicles are not in the scrotum at all. Can you tell me something about this problem?

Undescended testicles are quite frequently seen in male infants and may be unilateral (one side) or bilateral (both sides). In either case the majority will spontaneously descend by one year of age. If they do not, they will probably require surgical correction.

My child had an undescended testicle, which was operated on and brought down into the scrotum. Will it function normally?

If the other testicle is normal, whether or not it functions normally makes no difference, since one is all that is needed to ensure fertility. Psychologically, and from a cosmetic point of view, he will certainly be much better off having had the operation. It is a fascinating fact that in order to manufacture sperm, the testicles need the slightly cooler temperature of the scrotum, about two degrees lower than inside the abdomen.

My baby has a bulge on one side of the scrotum. What is it?

Chances are it is a hydrocele. This is an accumulation of fluid around the testicle; sometimes a hernia is present as well. Most of the time this fluid is gradually absorbed. The condition requires no treatment unless it persists past one year of age, and even then some will still spontaneously absorb.

My child just won't urinate. He hasn't wet in over eight hours. What shall I do?

If the infant or child is otherwise well and properly hydrated, the reason is usually some source of local discomfort around the urethra that produces pain on voiding, causing the child to hold back urine. You can sit him in a warm tub and let him void there since this frequently reduces the pain enough for him to relax. Virtually all children will void sooner or later but some may go as long as 24 hours. One should avoid catheterization (inserting a tube through the urethra in order to empty the bladder), since this is painful and will only add to the problem, as well as possibly introduce infection into the bladder if infection is not already present. Prolonged inability to void occurs extremely rarely, if at all, in children, so just be patient. Sooner or later he will produce.

6

Orthopedics

GENERAL

My child is double-jointed. Is this harmful?

Not at all. It often runs in families and is of no consequence except that he may be an outstanding gymnast.

What is an epiphysis?

This is the term used to denote the growth center of the bone. Growth centers are located near the ends of the long bones of the body. Fractures in children that involve this area need very careful orthopedic management in order to avoid, where possible, any impairment of growth of the affected bone.

POSTURE

How do I get him to stand up straight?

If his posture is really bad you should have your doctor take a good look at him to make sure there are no abnormalities. We are not only concerned with posture in profile but even more important from side to side—i.e., scoliosis. This is particularly true for children over ten years of age. In one study as many as 7 percent over the age of ten were found to have a significant deformity. If his physical examination is normal, the next step is to demonstrate good posture to the child. I usually will have him stand against the wall, shoulders and head touching the wall. I then ask him to place his back as tight to the wall as possible so there is not enough room to slide my hand between his back and the wall. He then walks forward in this position. Doing this exercise daily will remind him about his posture and is certainly a far better approach than nagging him constantly to stand up straight.

What is scoliosis?

It is a curvature of the spine, usually from side to side. It can be produced by a variety of conditions, but one of the most common is idiopathic scoliosis (cause unknown), which occurs most frequently in adolescent girls and which requires orthopedic treatment.

He looks swaybacked to me.

This is usually produced by a lumbar lordosis. This sway-back appearance with tummy stuck forward is common in most five to six-year-olds. Your doctor will check him out to make sure that the spine is straight and the hips are normal, which they usually are. No treatment for the condition is necessary and it will gradually correct with time.

WALKING AND SHOES

He is pigeon-toed. What should be done?

There are basically three conditions that cause toeing in.

First, where the front half of the foot (forefoot) is directed inward. This condition is quite frequent in infants. Sometimes there may even be a visible crease in the skin of the foot at the point of inward deviation. In this condition the foot has a C-shaped appearance. Some of these infants, especially those with a visible crease in the foot, will need some type of orthopedic correction. This can most often be accomplished by the use of a reverse-last shoe, but occasionally casts may be required. The infant's foot is so supple that a few weeks is all it generally takes.

The second cause for toeing in is the condition known as tibial torsion. The foot and knees are straight, but the tibia, or leg bone, rotates inward and gives the pigeon-toed appearance. Tibial torsion is very common and usually corrects itself by age five to six years. In an occasional severe case so-called Dennis-Brown splints may be used to aid correction. It reaches its maximum at age 18 to 20 months. Early walking may exaggerate the tendency but it certainly does *no* harm and therefore should not be the cause of any concern. Corrective shoes will not aid this condition.

The third condition which produces toeing in is called anteversion of the hip, or femoral torsion. The feet point inward, as do the knees. There is excessive inward rotation of the hips. These children often have a considerable amount of awkwardness and the condition is slow to correct but gradually improves up to about ten years of age. Many of these children have a habit of sitting with the legs splayed out, which further accentuates the internal rotation of the hip joint. Faulty sitting habits do not worsen the condition, but they do seem to make for a slower rate of improvement.

How can I tell if shoes fit properly?

There are two important things to check. First, make sure there is some space in front of the big toe; this you can feel with your thumb. Second, there should be no bulging on the outside of the foot. Always tend to err toward the large and not the small side. One inch too long, a half-inch too wide is a good rule to remember.

Are tennis shoes OK?

Tennis and other athletic shoes are perfectly all right as long as you can live with their appearance and at times the odor produced by excessive wear.

What is a Thomas heel?

This is a supportive device (wedge) that fits on the heel of the shoe and serves to bring heel extension up to the center of the arch, giving better support to the foot. This device gives comfort but does not correct the foot. Incidentally it can be quite helpful in adults as well.

Is it all right to let him wear his older brother's old shoes?

If the shoe fits, wear it! Yes, it is perfectly all right. Although it may disturb some people's sensibilities, it certainly helps the pocketbook.

What are cookies in the shoes?

These are small wedges placed in the shoes. For the most part they are of no help. They are probably indicated where the feet roll inward and the heels deviate outward, but this is really the only condition where they need to be used.

FRACTURES AND SPRAINS

What is a fracture?

A fracture is a disruption in the continuity of the bone. The term is synonymous with "break." The term greenstick fracture is used to denote a small crack in the shaft of the bone in children.

Is there any way I can tell at home if he has broken something? He always seems to be bumping into something and I hate to take him in each time.

Unfortunately, there is no way you can be sure there hasn't been a fracture. Experience is still probably the best teacher. However, if there is a lot of pain or a well-localized tenderness at one spot, chances are there is a break. Often you can sort things out a lot better after he's gotten over the initial shock of the fall or bump. After settling down and receiving comfort, he may surprise you by feeling fine. Persistence of pain and limitation of motion demand further attention.

I have heard that if you can walk on your foot it probably isn't fractured. Is this correct?

No, it's not. Even if you can move it fairly well it can still be broken, and it is always wise to check with your doctor.

What is best for the swelling produced by a sprain or bruise?

You should use cold compresses for the first 24 hours and warm compresses thereafter. The swelling is produced by bleeding in the soft tissues, and the cold constricts or narrows the blood vessels, preventing blood from leaking out from the damaged vessels.

OTHER PROBLEMS

What is Osgood-Schlatter disease?

This is a quite common condition in adolescent boys but can occur at a younger age too. It is thought to be caused by chronic trauma to the tibial area brought on by running, etc., and produces pain and swelling in the area just below and in front of the knee. You will want to have your doctor check to be sure about what it is. It is a benign condition and usually clears with limitation of activity.

My son has a small bump on the back of his hand. It has been there for quite some time and doesn't seem to bother him at all. What do you think it is?

It may well be a ganglion but you will want to check with your doctor. If it is a ganglion, it will probably go away on its own, but may take months to do so. These are small cysts of the tendon sheaths or linings and they occur most freqeuntly around the wrist, back of the knee, and the top of the foot. They are benign and almost never need to be removed. They are also known as Bible cysts since in the good old days a slam with the family Bible got rid of them for good!

My six-year-old awakened this morning complaining of pain in the neck, but otherwise seems well. What should I do?

You will want to check with your doctor but chances are this is a condition known as *acute torticollis*. It is not associated with any symptoms of illness, nor usually with a history of any injury, but just comes on spontaneously. Most often a peculiar sleeping position causes the neck muscles to go into painful spasm. The head is usually tilted slightly to one side and the child is unable, without considerable pain, to turn the head to the side or to look upward, but is usually able to bend the chin down. Heat and aspirin are the treatment needed to resolve the condition in 24 to 48 hours. The child needn't remain in bed and can be encouraged to move around as much as he can tolerate.

Does anything need to be done about webbed feet?

This condition is known as *syndactyly*. If the toes are aligned properly, and in most cases they are, nothing need be done. Webbing or syndactyly of the fingers is a more unusual condition and surgical correction is required to achieve proper function.

I have noticed that his toes overlap. Is this a condition that needs correction?

Overlapping of the toes, usually the third and fourth toe, is seen fairly often in infants and is of no significance. It often runs in families and there is no need to do anything about it.

He has flat feet. What should I do?

Before the age of two it is difficult to tell if the feet will really be flat because of the amount of fat on the sole of the foot. This makes virtually all infants' feet appear to be flat. Two types of flat feet persist. By far the more common is the flat foot that frequently runs in families, causes no trouble, and can be forgotten. Some of the best athletes I have seen have flat feet. The other is the rigid flat foot that will not bend properly; in this case there may well be a bone abnormality and this type of foot should be evaluated by the orthopedist.

My child has knock-knees. What can be done about this?

"Knock-knee" is caused by an inward rotation of the thighbone, or femur, and is thus referred to as *femoral torsion*. As mentioned elsewhere there may be associated toeing in as well. Children with this condition often tend to be a bit more awkward than most. This condition usually self-corrects with time.

7

Cardiovascular System

HEART DISEASE

What can be done to prevent heart disease from developing?
Identification of the high-risk child is of great importance. In cases of abnormally high blood fats, treatment is already available. In general, emphasis on guarding against excessive caloric intake and the ingestion of too much cholesterol is certainly of great importance and should be a part of routine well-baby care. Long-term studies as to the effect of dietary changes in children on the development of heart disease are not yet available but just about everybody agrees that eating in moderation is a good idea, as is a general decrease in the amount of saturated animal fat.

Do the risk factors that apply for adults as far as heart disease is concerned also apply to children? Could you list them?
Yes, the risk factors very definitely apply to children and are going to receive far more attention in the coming years. They include: elevation of blood pressure; smoking; obesity—not by itself but in association with high blood pressure; elevation of blood cholesterol and or triglycerides; family history of onset of coronary artery disease under age 50; and too much stress, which is just as applicable to the child as it is to the adult.

What is the incidence of elevated blood cholesterol in children?
I don't think we really know at present since this is some-

thing which has only recently begun to receive attention. In some series as many as 1 in 500 seem to have a level high enough to warrant treatment with diet and/or medication in the hopes of preventing heart disease at a later date.

What about restricting the amount of cholesterol in my child's diet? Do you think that this is a good idea?

We still have no proof that lowering the blood cholesterol will prevent the development of heart disease, although there is no doubt that elevated cholesterol is a proven risk factor. The only exception is the Type 2 familial elevation of cholesterol, which does show up in childhood and should be treated by proper dietary restrictions. Most experts now feel that overeating in any form is probably just as important in the development of heart disease. Restriction of cholesterol in the infant's diet may have serious effects since cholesterol is very important in the development of the nervous system. It's significant that breast milk contains very high levels of cholesterol, proving its importance for your baby. What we badly need is an ongoing study such as that done by the NIH in Framingham, Mass., but devoted to the accumulation of data in children, not adults. As of this writing, however, it is not felt to be a sound idea to restrict cholesterol in the average child's diet; on the other hand ingestion of large amounts of cholesterol and also of total calories is certainly to be discouraged.

How do you feel about exercise for children?

This may sound like a silly question and yet I have been asked it on numerous occasions. I think exercise is of the greatest importance for the developing child and of equal importance later in maintaining health. It amazes me to see the number of children who lead sedentary lives and I decry the situation that exists in most schools, particularly the public schools, where almost no attention is devoted to the development of good physical-fitness habits. We pay all kinds of attention to diet, dental care, immunizations, all of which have proven preventive value to the child, and yet we are still ignorant about exercise. Every child should have the opportunity to participate in physical activities but, more importantly, should be taught the kind of activities he will be able to use lifelong. These should become as habitual as brushing the teeth. Team sports are great, but over the long haul, other forms of exercise such as biking, running, tennis, swimming, and the like will stand him in better stead. You, as parents, set the standards for your children, so make sure you pay attention to this area both by talking about it and also by participating in some form of exercise as a family unit. This doesn't mean that you have to jog 20 miles every morning, but taking a walk or perhaps riding bikes together on a regular basis can have great value in emphasizing exercise as an important part of family life.

Should my child have his blood pressure taken, and if so at what age should this first be done?

He definitely should have his blood pressure checked, as hypertension does occur in children. Most pediatricians usually begin at two to three years of age and repeat the measurement at each examination thereafter. As some of the newer instruments for obtaining blood pressure accurately and easily in infants become more available, we will probably begin even earlier.

What is the incidence of congenital heart disease?

Approximately 8 infants per 1000 born have some form of congenital heart disease. This statistic has not changed in the past 15 years.

What about risk factors that you can identify early?

Three important ways to identify the high-risk child are to evaluate premature onset of heart disease in the family, measure elevation of blood lipids (fats) in the family, and routinely measure blood pressure in children.

What is the most common type of congenital heart disease?

Ventricular septal defect (VSD) is the most common heart defect at birth and accounts for approximately 25 percent of all cases. The outlook for this condition is usually good since many VSDs will close spontaneously in time and many more have a tendency to get smaller with age.

What is meant by cardiac catheterization?

Tubes are inserted into the blood vessels and heart in order to take pressure measurements and visualize various parts of the circulatory system. This technique may be applied to babies who are only a few hours old and, in skilled hands, is not only a safe but an extremely accurate tool in the diagnosis of congenital heart disease.

How early can cardiac surgery be done?

Immediately after birth if required. The advances in this field are tremendous and continue unabated, so that the child born with congenital heart disease today has a far better chance of survival and a full life than ever before.

MURMURS AND OTHER CONDITIONS

My doctor told me on my child's recent examination that he has a functional heart murmur. What is it and what implications does it have?

A functional murmur occurs in as many as 50 percent of children. It is a soft "swishing" sound heard in conjunction with the heartbeat and is produced by the flow of the blood through the normal heart. This type of murmur is entirely innocent; there is absolutely nothing wrong with the heart. There is no need for any further study and no need for any restriction of activity or for any concern. Most go away in time. (The reason that children usually outgrow them is that although the sound is still present it no longer can be heard because of the growth in the size of the chest and the change in the chest configuration with age.) Even if they do not go away, they are still of no significance. Your pediatrician mentioned it to you so that if someone else spotted it somewhere you would know it was there and of no concern.

My child was told that he has a murmur and therefore he should not do strenuous exercise or engage in competitive athletics. What do you think?

Since the overwhelming majority of murmurs in children are innocent, as just indicated, I strongly believe that no child should be restricted from any activity on the basis of heart disease until he has had the benefit of a thorough evaluation by a cardiologist who is familiar with the problems of children.

What percentage of murmurs heard in children are innocent?
Ninety-five percent fall into this category.

My baby has some blueness around the mouth at times, and occasionally his hands and feet turn blue. I have read so much about blue babies. Does this sound abnormal?
No, it does not. This type of blueness results from some vascular immaturity in the baby. Real cyanosis or blueness of the kind we worry about will invariably involve the tongue. So if the tongue is pink and the baby appears otherwise healthy it is of no concern.

My child complained of chest pain the other day. What should I do?
You will want to check with your doctor but chances are that this is what we call chest-wall pain. It is almost always of muscular origin, usually brought on by a lot of physical activity, often exaggerated by deep breathing or movement. Complaints of chest pain in childhood are not uncommon. Chest pain of cardiac origin has the same characteristics in the child as in the adult except that, of course, it is very rare in children.

My 13-year-old daughter fainted last Sunday while in church. Is this serious?
The classic fainting spell usually occurs in the teen-age girl on a hot day while in a crowded, poorly ventilated area. There is also frequently a family history of fainting spells. The episode is usually of brief duration and the child returns to normal immediately on arousing. You will, of course, want your doctor to be aware of the event and to relate the story to him. One kind of fainting we do worry about occurs in association with exercise since it could possibly mean that it was caused by some abnormal heart rhythm. But the majority of episodes fall into the "no need for concern" category.

8

Ear, Nose, and Throat

HEARING

When should he have his hearing tested?

All children should have some sort of formal audiometric screening done. By the time he is three years of age a reasonably accurate test can be performed, at least for screening purposes.

What is the most common cause of hearing loss?

Wax in the ears.

You mentioned that for the young infant observation is still the best method of evaluating hearing. What about as he gets a bit older?

By eight months of age we can condition him to respond to various sounds. For example, a piercing sound may be associated with a pleasant visual response. One can be very accurate using this method.

By two and a half to three years of age play audiometry can be done, which consists of conditioning the child to various social sounds.

By four and half to five we can begin to do the classical screening audiometry. This is an average; in some children we can get some accuracy on an audiogram as young as two years of age.

Can loud noise injure my child's hearing?

There is a good deal of concern about the level of environmental noise to which we all are exposed and its possible deleterious effects, both psychological and physical. To date there are no firm conclusions to be drawn. It is reasonable, however, if the child will be frequently exposed to very loud noise, for example, if he plays in the local rock group, to fit him with protective earplugs.

He seems to shout so much. Do you suppose he could be having difficulty hearing?

Almost never does a hearing impairment manifest itself by loud talking. It's just a common childhood habit but may be accentuated by his copying adults, so watch yourself! People with conductive hearing loss frequently tend to talk more softly rather than the opposite.

My child received a severe blow to the ear. Is it likely to harm his hearing?

A boxing-type blow to the ear can frequently produce a rupture or break of the eardrum.There is usually sudden pain, but even without this symptom you will want to check with your physician.

EARS—GENERAL

He occasionally says he feels dizzy. Is it likely to be an ear problem?

Dizzy spells are far less likely to be produced by ear problems in children than in adults. Other causes are more frequent.

My doctor frequently mentions that my child has some fluid in the ear. What does this mean?

He is referring to a condition known as serious otitis media, in which there is an accumulation of fluid behind the middle eardrum. This is usually caused by an ear infection, but it can persist following the infection or at times arise spontaneously. Usually the older child will complain of a sense of fullness or stuffiness in the ears and frequently you will notice a hearing loss. This condition seems to be on the increase and we are not certain why. Infections, allergy, and perhaps other as yet poorly understood factors are responsible. Most of the time the fluid goes away spontaneously and does no harm. However, if it persists, it seems to make the child more susceptible to ear infections and it may damage the ear, although we are not sure of this. In cases where the fluid does seem to persist or recur your doctor will probably want to look into the situation further.

What about these tubes in the ears? What do they do?

In children with persistent or chronic fluid in the middle ear the fluid may be permanently drained into the external canal by means of a small polyethylene tube inserted through the eardrum.

He has a bug in his ear. What shall I do?

Pour a little alcohol in the ear canal. This will usually produce a rapid demise of the insect. Even a bit of gin will do just fine. Lacking this, you can use plain water and, unless the bug is a good swimmer, this will accomplish the same purpose.

He has a berry in his ear. What should I do?

Don't try to get it out. You will succeed only in pushing it further down the ear canal and probably just cause him further discomfort. It is best to let the doctor do it since with special instruments designed for the purpose it is usually not difficult.

Do you approve of piercing the ears, and if so who should do it?

I used to think that it should only be done by a physician but in recent years have changed my mind since there are many stores where it can be safely done by *trained* personnel. I would make sure, however, that it will be carefully done under sterile conditions. Don't forget to use gold to keep the ears open as it seldom causes any local skin irritation.

My child has a tendency to accumulate wax in the ears and often complains that he is uncomfortable. What can I do about this?

Most of the time I leave wax in the ear canals alone, partically in the infant who is perfectly happy. You may use a Q-tip to clean around the outside of the ear canal but do not attempt to clean inside since the ear canal is very sensitive and can easily be injured. Besides, it usually does not bother him anyway! It is supposed to be there and performs a valuable function in lubricating the canal, protecting the ear from infection and trapping foreign material. Occasionally it can cause difficulty and you should check with your physician to see how he manages this problem. Mostly, we prescribe ear drops that will dissolve the wax and couple this with some gentle irrigation of the ear canals with room-temperature water dispensed by an ear syringe that you can buy at the drugstore. Your doctor can show you how the procedure can be done at home. This is not something that needs to be done frequently. Rarely the wax may be hard and impacted and need to be removed by an ear specialist.

Colds, Nosebleeds, Etc.

He has a cold. Can he go on the plane?

I think it is reasonable to let him. I have seen no difficulty with pressure changes. If he is very "stopped up," a decongestant prescribed by your pediatrician might prove helpful.

Why does he get nosebleeds?

The most frequent reason is excessive dryness of the nasal membrane, which is produced by dry air in the wintertime, particularly forced-air heat. Allergy is also an important contributing factor since it can keep the nasal membranes in an irritated and congested state. Recurrent nosebleeds need to be checked, but usually nothing serious is found. Prolonged bleeding may mean an underlying clotting defect and will have to be evaluated further. Humidification of the inside air in winter is an important preventive measure, as is some simple lubricant such as Borafax or Vaseline.

How do you stop a nosebleed?

The best way is to hold the tip of the nose, squeezing the nostrils gently but firmly together. Continue this for 15 to 20 minutes. Since most nosebleeds occur in the septum or middle of the nose, well up toward the front, this simple maneuver will stop at least 95 percent of the nosebleeds in children. Cold compresses over the bridge of the nose or ice bags on the forehead are no help. If a child tends to have nosebleeds, one can practice the maneuver and assure him by demonstrating that he will be able to breathe through his mouth quite comfortably.

He put something up his nose. How shall I get it out?

Unless it is right at the tip, and unless you are the confident type with previous experience in such matters, best leave it alone, as you will only make the doctor's job more difficult.

Why does his nose run?

There are mucous glands lining the nose that produce mucus. This is a protective substance which defends the body against infection as well as inhaled foreign substances. Changes in temperature, and infection and allergy all can stimulate these glands to secrete more than the normal amount of liquid. This excessive mucus runs out of the front of the nose and some of it drips down the back of the nose into the throat (postnasal drip), where it is swallowed. This is the normal mechanism by which the body rids itself of this fluid. A postnasal drip is really a runny nose; only it is running in a different direction.

He has a lot of discharge from just one side of his nose.

Persistent thick yellowish discharge from only one nostril is frequently associated with a very foul odor and is almost always indicative of a foreign body that the child has inserted up the nose. He should be checked carefully by your doctor. Do not attempt to remove it yourself as you will only suceed in frightening or injuring him, and pushing it farther up the nose, making the job much more difficult. Leave it to the professional.

THROAT—TONSILS AND ADENOIDS

My child frequently gets hoarse. What causes it?

Occasionally children will develop hoarseness from vocal abuse. It occurs more frequently in boys, and occasionally continued vocal abuse will produce actual nodules on the vocal cords. This condition should be checked with your physician but usually correction of the bad habit and the passage of time cures the problem.

What do the tonsils do?

They are composed of so-called lymphatic tissue, which is very important in the production of antibodies that fight infection in the body. Other aggregates of this tissue include the adenoids and lymph nodes.

What is tonsillitis? Are there different kinds?

Tonsillitis refers to an inflammation or infection of the tonsils (the two large pieces of tissue in the back of the throat). Many different bacteria and viruses can cause tonsillitis and the term does not identify which infecting agent is at fault. For example, one may have a tonsillitis caused by a streptococcus, staphylococcus, or any one of a number of viruses. The term *pharyngitis* is often used to cover all infections of the throat, including infection of the tonsils.

Are there any reasons to take the tonsils out?

Yes, I believe that on occasion removal of the tonsils is indicated. Some children develop repeated infections that are well localized in the tonsils and are frequently caused by strep throat. Even though these patients are given antibiotics to eradicate the infection, they just never seem to really clear up between episodes. As a result they miss a great deal of school, they never really seem up to par, their appetite is poor, and they go from one infection to the next. In these situations removal of the tonsils may frequently be of great help. Very rarely, the tonsillar tissue is so large that it actually makes breathing difficult, and when the tissue is inflamed and swollen it produces further difficulty. In this situation removal of the tonsils is definitely indicated.

If the tonsils are big does it mean that they are more likely to cause problems?

No, it does not. The tonsillar tissue is present at birth but undergoes a gradual increase in size until it reaches its maximum around five to six years of age. Thereafter the tonsils gradually shrink so that in most adults they are quite small. It is usually the five-year-old who is thought to have "big tonsils," but as you see, this is all part of normal development.

What are the adenoids?

They are pieces of lymphatic tissue that are situated in the nasopharynx, the area up behind the back of the throat. If you were to walk along the tongue you would come to the uvula, that little piece of tissue that hangs down in the middle of the throat. If you took another couple of steps and looked straight up you would look into the area of the nasopharynx, where the back of the nose and mouth connect. This is a rather difficult area to visualize and it is impossible to see the adenoids without using a special mirror. Another method of examination is to reach back and up with the finger to feel the tissue. Technically there are some other pieces of adenoid tissue as well, but for practical purposes when one speaks of adenoids it refers to these.

He snores at night.

This is usually caused by enlarged adenoidal tissue, which results in obstruction of airflow through the nose. Frequently there is associated mouth breathing as well, which is noticeable in the daytime, and there may or may not be frequent ear infections. The adenoids may be enlarged on the basis of chronic infection in the tissue but allergy is also a common cause, and the situation will need to be evaluated by your doctor.

Do the adenoids ever have to be removed?

Yes, on occasion they create problems. They can be so large as to obstruct the flow of air through the nose, causing mouth breathing, snoring at night, and nasal speech. Because this tissue is located near the opening of the Eustachian tubes (small canals that lead from the middle ear to the nose) it may sometimes block this connection, which is thought to be a contributory factor in producing middle-ear infections in some children. These are two situations where their removal may be justified, providing the child has been carefully evaluated by both the pediatrician

Doctor's Call Hour

and the ear, nose, and throat surgeon. There are some children who benefit by the removal of both tonsils and adenoids simultaneously. I would like to stress, however, that the number of children who need their tonsils and/or adenoids removed is quite small.

9

Eyes

When should my child have his eyes checked and who should perform the examination?

Every child should be given the benefit of a complete eye examination by an ophthalmologist (a medical doctor who specializes in eye problems) sometime during early childhood, four to five years of age. By this time he is usually old enough to cooperate in a complete examination. If his eyes are normal this examination will usually suffice for the remainder of the childhood years. Color vision, depth perception, fusion, and a screen for amblyopia, or lazy eye, are all part of this evaluation.

Beginning at age three, all children should receive some type of visual screening at their routine yearly physical examination. If there is a family history of eye problems, especially on both sides of the family, an examination at a younger age by an ophthalmologist is important. By the time he is six months of age he is old enough for a reasonably thorough eye examination.

What is amblyopia?

Amblyopia, or "lazy eye," as it is frequently called, occurs in approximately 2 percent of the population. In this condition there is a muscle imbalance of the two eyes and images of an object are projected on nonidentical points of the retina. In order to avoid double vision one of these images is usually suppressed by the brain. This eventually leads to deterioration of vision in that eye. If diagnosed early, the condition can almost always be corrected.

Are headaches frequently the result of eye problems?

Despite what is frequently said, headaches are almost never caused by eye problems—so look for a cause elsewhere. One exception might be severe myopia (nearsightedness), which is usually apparent by observing the child.

GLASSES

Are sunglasses all right to wear? He loves to play with them.

They are perfectly all right to use and will not harm the eyes.

Will wearing glasses make his eyes weaker?

No, it won't and usually he will want to wear glasses since he will find them so helpful.

Is there such a thing as a child being too young for glasses?

No, if he needs them he can wear them at virtually any age. In addition, contact lenses can frequently be used with great success in young children.

EYE PROBLEMS

He got something in his eye. What should I do?

Rinse with copious amounts of plain water. If this doesn't remove the foreign body pull the lower lid down and, if you can see the speck of dirt or whatever, dab it with a clean handkerchief or tissue. If it is not visible, pull the upper lid down, holding it firmly but gently by the eyelashes, depress it gently with a Q-tip or match, then pull it up over the match to expose the under surface and again dab it off. There is often a sensation of something still being in the eye for a few minutes but this should quickly go away. If the child continues to complain consult your doctor. It is a good idea to practice this maneuver with the upper lid before an occasion arises where you need to do it.

Something splashed in his eye. What should I do?

Immediately wash his face and eye with copious amounts of plain cool tap water for five to ten minutes. If there then appears to be inflammation (redness) of the eye or he complains of pain, you should check with your doctor.

What is pinkeye?

Just another term for conjunctivitis, which means an inflammation of the lining of the eye; it usually results in a pink color in the white of the eye. Many times conjunctivitis is associated with a viral illness and no specific treatment is necessary but you will want to consult your doctor. If the conjunctivitis is bilateral (both sides) it is often viral in origin and may clear promptly. Some warm compresses several times a day will relieve local discomfort. If it is only on one side, and especially if there is a thick yellowish-green discharge, it is probably bacterial and will require antibiotics to clear it up. Let your doctor decide which treatment is indicated.

GENERAL

Can reading too much harm the eyes?

For the most part, no.

Will reading in poor light harm the eyes?

Contrary to popular belief it won't harm them, although it is not a habit to be encouraged if for no other reason than the obvious one that you can't see as well.

Will bright colors aid in developing the eyes?

I am sure he will enjoy a multicolored and interesting environment, but as far as we know, bright colors will not increase his visual capacities.

I noticed that he likes to hold things close to him. Is he nearsighted?

Most infants and young children will hold things close to them for visual inspection. First, they seem to get much more out of the experience psychologically since theirs is a smaller world than that of adults. In addition, they have tremendous accommodating powers. That is to say, their eye muscles, being new and strong, will actually magnify the object greatly and they therefore enjoy doing it. Physiologically the young child is actually farsighted (hyperopic) and can therefore see better at a distance, but for these two reasons he actually prefers to have whatever he is looking at close to him.

His eyes are crossed. Will he outgrow it?

All babies show some tendency to cross the eyes under three months of age. This is of no concern unless there is a consistent deviation of the eye in one direction, which is abnormal at any age and should be evaluated by the ophthalmologist as soon as the condition is diagnosed. It will not go away spontaneously.

Will eye surgery to straighten the eyes affect his ability to read?

No, it will not.

10

Teeth

DENTAL CARE—GENERAL

Why is it so important to take care of the primary teeth?

First of all, the good dental habits you instill in the child will, one hopes, continue when he has his permanent teeth. Also, these teeth are important in ensuring adequate bone growth and proper development of the dental arch that will hold the permanent teeth. Inadequate growth, as well as asymmetrical growth secondary to prematurely lost deciduous (baby) teeth, can be a significant problem.

At what age should he begin to brush his teeth?

When he is a toddler he can begin by using a *soft* brush or prior to this you may even use a bit of gauze on the finger. Do not use toothpaste at this age since most young children do not like it and it is not necessary anyway. The important thing is to introduce him to brushing early and to make it enjoyable for him. The earlier the habit is formed the better. Although brushing the teeth can be started when he is a toddler, cleaning the teeth should begin after eruption of the first tooth, with a piece of gauze on the finger.

Is there any way to help him brush? I find it very difficult?

The ideal position is to stand behind him with his chin cupped gently in your left hand so that the child looks up and backwards at you. Your right hand is free to brush. This is a physically close and affectionate position and is far better than reaching out with the child standing opposite you.

I wonder if it is all right if my children use the mechanical water-pulsating tooth-cleaning devices?

I think that they are permissible for the older child, but only with careful parental supervision. If used in an unsupervised manner the force of the water jet can do a great deal of damage to the gum tissue. If your child is maintaining proper dental hygiene and your dentist feels that his teeth and gum tissue are in good shape, it will not be necessary to use any sort of mechanical device.

How often should the teeth be brushed?

You should let the child brush once a day. The parents of a young child should brush his teeth once a day. By the time he is five he may brush twice daily on his own but you should check to make sure he is doing an adequate job. Of course thorough brushing after each meal is the ideal but it is not easy to achieve.

What kind of toothpaste should he use?

One approved by the American Dental Association that contains fluoride.

Should my child use dental floss?

Yes, he certainly should; your dentist will be glad to instruct him in its use.

Should I use fluoride?

Definitely. Most areas of the country have fluoridated water, but check with the local health department if you are in doubt. If you are using well water have it analyzed. The health department will do this without charge, as well as a bacterial count. Water added to the formula in a fluoridated area is sufficient and in breast-fed babies enough is transmitted in breast milk to meet the baby's requirements. If needed, fluoride drops may be prescribed by your doctor.

How shall we go about choosing a dentist for our child?

Most dentists graduating today have had far more training in the area of children's dentistry (or pedodontics, as it is called) than their older counterparts. Many excellent general dentists can deal effectively with young children. One who shows interest in children, who is gentle, and who takes the time required is the kind that you will want.

When should my child see the dentist for the first time?

The first formal visit to the dentist should occur after all the primary teeth have erupted. Somewhere around three years of age is an ideal time. At this first visit your dentist will probably want to take some X-rays of the teeth and do some light cleaning and polishing.

How often should he see the dentist?

At six-month intervals. There are two high-risk periods in the child. One is five to seven years of age, at which time caries can become a very serious problem, and the other is the teen-age period. These are times of rapid metabolic changes and also times where bad eating habits are particularly prevalent.

How do you feel about routine dental X-rays in children?

I believe that the advantages outweigh the risks, but this does not mean that they should be used without careful thought and supervision. Important safeguards include use of high-speed film, proper shielding, careful focusing of the beam, and good developing techniques so that the film will not have to be retaken, choosing views that are easily obtained in children and therefore won't have to be retaken. Some of the things found include supernumerary teeth, cysts, and tumors. When teeth are injured fractures of the root may be seen.

Are there any medications that can damage the teeth?

Tetracycline is an antibiotic that should not be used in children under eight years of age because it can permanently stain the teeth even in small doses and even if given for only a very short period of time.

His "baby" teeth look crooked. What should be done about them?

The lower central incisors often appear rotated when they first erupt but asymmetries in deciduous teeth or any problem with malalignment that *persists* is very unusual and needs further investigation.

DENTAL ACCIDENTS

My three-year-old fell and loosened his two upper front teeth. What should be done?

He should be seen by the dentist. The teeth may be splinted in order to help them remain in place. An X-ray may also be a good idea in order to check the integrity of the roots of the teeth and to see if there is any damage to the underlying permanent teeth that have not yet erupted.

What should be done if the teeth are driven up into the gum by a hard fall?

This is a frequent type of injury and is best handled by letting things alone. Deciduous teeth will almost always reerupt and move back down into their normal position. This type of injury usually involves the upper central incisors. The situation is far more serious for permanent teeth, as they will not re-erupt and will need to be brought down into proper position.

What should I do if one of the teeth is knocked out?

If a deciduous tooth, your dentist will probably not attempt to reimplant it since most will abscess and eventually be lost anyway. It is important to take the tooth along with your child since the dentist will want to inspect it to make sure that it is the whole tooth and that part or all of the root is not still in place. If it is, he will want to remove it and may take an X-ray to be sure.

If a permanent tooth, it should be considered an emergency and the tooth should be wrapped in a damp tissue and taken immediately to the nearest dentist. Time is of the essence and the faster the tooth can be reimplanted the better the chances of the procedure being successful.

What if he knocks a permanent tooth out and we are not near dental help?

Wash the tooth carefully in a salt-water solution (one teaspoon of salt in one pint water) and immediately place it firmly into the socket, making sure that the proper surface is facing outward. Then make your way to the dentist. The chances of successful reimplantation are much better by doing this than by waiting several hours for dental help.

My three-year-old fell and bumped his upper front tooth a few weeks ago. I have noticed that it now looks somewhat gray. What does this mean?

It means that the circulation to the tooth has been impaired and the tooth is dying. As long as it seems stable and is not loose it may remain in until it falls out by itself. No attempt should be made to remove it.

ORTHODONTIA

What is the reason for orthodontic treatment. Is it really necessary?

Correction of various spacing and positional abnormalities of the teeth in order to produce a more perfect bite means there is a much better chance of the teeth remaining in a healthy condition. Just like any machine, the smoother the teeth work the longer they last. Aesthetics also play a major role in the need for orthodontia. The "buck-toothed" child not only has a mechanical abnormality of his bite but perhaps more important is the detrimental psychological effect his appearance is going to have on him as he gets older.

Do children usually accept orthodontia fairly easily?

Yes, they do, and most orthodontists work well with the children on a one-to-one basis with a minimum of parental involvement. Another factor that makes the whole thing easier is that we are now into a second generation of orthodontic care. Many parents have been through it themselves, realize that it is not all that traumatic, and are convinced of its value.

What is the success rate of orthodontia?

In about 80 percent of the cases there is correction of the dental malalignment as well as cosmetic improvement. In the 20 percent group, there is some improvement, which may or may not be permanent, and in a few cases, orthodontia may not be successful.

At what age can my child start with the orthodontist?

He can start as young as 6 or 7 years of age but the average is 10 to 12 for girls and 11 to 13 years for boys, since, of course, they develop later.

How long does the treatment take on the average?

The average duration of therapy is two to four years.

Do these dental abnormalities tend to run in families?

Yes, there is strong hereditary influence; if you needed orthodontia the chances are very high that your children will.

Are the effects of orthodontia limited to the teeth?

No, they are not. It will often have a very favorable effect on the developing contour of the facial bones as well and thus greatly improve the appearance of the child in future years.

What is the incidence of children who require orthodontic treatment?

It is estimated that as many as 65 to 70 percent of children would benefit from it.

How do I know if my orthodontist is fully trained and certified?

If he is a member of the American Association of Orthodontics you can be sure he has met all the requirements.

It seems as though all my daughter's friends are talking about head gear. What is this device anyway?

It is an appliance used by orthodontists to help control and redirect growth as well as to actually move teeth. Approximately 75 percent of children who need orthodontic treatment are going to need head gear at some point. With increasing usage the child already has many friends who are using it and usually quickly adapts. Most frequently it need only be worn during sleep. In my experience it is a remarkably effective device.

My two-year-old grinds his teeth at night. Is this serious?

Certainly not. Incidentally, bruxism, as teeth grinding is called, does not mean that your child is infested with worms. There are discomforts associated with eruption and spacing of teeth in phases of rapid growth which can make them uncomfortable at times and be a factor in teeth grinding. It is also more likely to occur in the tense child. There is no specific treatment and it is almost always self-limited and causes no harm.

My dentist has advised that my child have several teeth pulled in order to make room for the others. Does this sound correct?

Yes, it does. It is frequently better to have, for example, 28 teeth that are well positioned than 32 which are "jumbled" and otherwise malaligned.

My three-year-old sucks his thumb. Does this mean that he is going to need orthodontia?

Thumb-sucking from three to six years of age is of no concern to the orthodontist. If it is prolonged past that time (after the permanent teeth begin coming in, especially the upper central incisors), then it can produce deformity. In the vast majority of cases the child has stopped the habit before this time.

11

Skin

GENERAL

What are some general rules about good skin care?

Resist the temptation to anoint the skin constantly with powders and creams.

Avoid excessive bathing of your child (he will be thrilled), especially in winter.

Avoid excessive exposure to sun.

Don't use bubble bath preparations, as they frequently produce allergic skin eruptions.

Excessively prolonged bathing causes overhydration of the skin, which is followed by evaporation and excessive dehydration, all of which contributes to excessive dryness and irritation. Beware the boat floater who may remain immersed for an hour or two.

Proper humidification is especially important in the winter since dry, warm air increases the amount of water loss from the skin through evaporation.

Dry the infant and young child after bathing and be sure to pay attention to the skin fold areas such as under the arms where moisture tends to accumulate and produce rashes.

My child's skin is so dry. Is there anything I can do about it?

Reduced water content, not oil, causes dry skin in many children and adults and usually nothing needs to be done about it. In the winter the child is inside for long periods of time and exposed to dry, warm air in which the humidity may be as low as 15 percent. This warm, dry air evaporates what little moisture there is in the skin and therefore leads to further drying. The same is true with frequent bathing, which leads to further evaporation of moisture after the bath is completed. You can cut down somewhat in this area; how much depends on your aesthetic and olfactory sensibilities. Quick showers are a good idea. In addition you can also buy a humidifier, which will add considerable moisture to the air. Many can be attached to the central heating system. Dryness of the air is particularly a problem in those homes with forced-air heating. Some lotions can be helpful. Finally, avoid soap and detergents and try one of the several soap substitutes available.

SUN EXPOSURE

What can I do about sunburn?

Once you have gotten it there's little to be done. The tissues of the skin have been damaged, and it's just a matter of time healing them. Usually some sort of topical cream to shield the skin from the air will give relief. However, if there is blistering the burn may need some type of dressing and your doctor should be consulted. If severe generalized sunburn has occurred, the child may have fever and become seriously ill; your physician should be consulted at once.

How do you feel about sun exposure for children?

There is no doubt that sunlight is an important factor in the development of skin cancer. But each of us has a certain amount of time our skin can be exposed to the ultraviolet radiation of the sun before it causes damage. You might call this total sun time. This total must be spread over a lifetime, and if it is mostly used up during the childhood years there isn't going to be much left for later. Thus exposing the children constantly is not a good idea. For the red-headed, fair-skinned child who freckles easily it can be especially dangerous. The use of various sun screens, those that contain PABA (para-aminobenzoic acid), is certainly a good idea if your child will be exposed on a prolonged basis. He will "tan," but it may take him the summer to do so, which, according to current thinking, may be just the way it should be done. The very fair-skinned individual may need a sun block, one of the preparations that almost totally excludes the sun's damaging effects.

We may well be on the threshold of an age where that healthy tan is no longer the "in" thing, although the feeling of well-being many people experience when tanning in the sun makes it unlikely that we will ever see an end to the sun worshiper. What we will see, however, and I think what the child should be taught, is that just like anything else—too much of a good thing is too much.

ACNE

What causes acne?

Obstruction of the sebaceous ducts in the skin produces a backup of the oily, sebaceous material that results in the "pimples" of acne.

Is diet an important factor in aggravating acne?

Probably not in the majority of people, but there are certain individuals who react adversely to chocolate, nuts, and soft drinks, and their skin is certainly made worse by their ingestion. With the cooperation of your teen-ager you should be able to tell if he falls into this group. If not, there seems to be no need for diet restriction.

OTHER SKIN PROBLEMS

I notice that my four-year-old has a small area on the scalp where she is losing her hair. What causes this?

You will want to take her in to be checked. The diagnosis may be trichotillomania, a fancy name for hair pulling. The child pulls out the hair, often when drowsy or during sleep, and is usually unobserved by the parents. Usually the hairs in the area of

loss are of different sizes and some are corkscrew-shaped because
of excessive twisting. This is a self-limited condition and nothing
need be done about it. In time the hair will grow back.

My child has warts. What should I do about them?
Wish them away! Don't laugh; whether or not the power of
suggestion or the passage of time makes them go away, I'm not
sure, but it works. Occasionally, one that is causing pain or
discomfort because it's on the foot or finger may need some
treatment, but even these are best left alone if possible.

What about moles? My child seems to have quite a few of them.
They are usually of no significance and begin to appear at
age three or even earlier and increase in frequency at puberty.
Moles (or nevi, as they are called) seldom cause any trouble unless they are of an unusual variety or undergo some change in
size, deepening of color, or change in texture.

**I have noticed that my teen-age daughter has a lot of stretch
marks on her skin, especially around the hips. Will these go
away?**
These are much more likely to occur in very fair-skinned
individuals, particularly those who tend to be overweight. They
will usually not go away.

My child gets a lot of cold sores. What can I do about them?
These are caused by the herpes virus. Recurrent cold sores
can be triggered by sun, elevation in body temperature, emotional
stress, aspirin, and occasionally trauma. There is no specific
treatment other than some topical creams for discomfort and
even these are seldom necessary. They last on the average of
8 to 12 days and go away on their own.

What is swimmer's itch?
It is an itchy eruption of the skin caused by the schistosome,
a tiny parasite found in fresh water in areas where pollution is a
problem. The condition is self-limited and stays localized to the
skin. A topical ointment like A & D is often helpful.

What can I do if my child is stung by a jellyfish?

Jellyfish or sea nettle bites respond well to meat tenderizer applied locally. The papain in the meat tenderizer digests the foreign protein material from the jellyfish, minimizing the sting.

I notice that he always seems to have a red area of skin around the corner of the mouth. Is it an allergy or what?

Most always it is from the habit of licking the skin around the mouth. Saliva in and of itself is irritating to the skin and, coupled with the drying effect produced by constant evaporation, can be very irritating and produce this red ringlike area. Pointing out to the child that this is the cause of the problem frequently cures the habit as the skin is usually dry, "cracky," and a source of discomfort to him. A little Vaseline helps.

12

Allergies

What causes allergy?

The basic problem is hyperreactivity of tissue. When certain people are stimulated by dust, foods, etc., their body cells have a tendency to overreact and produce the symptoms we associate with allergy. These symptoms include runny nose, watery eyes, skin rashes, and wheezing, to mention some of the best known. It is interesting to note that in addition to allergy other factors such as infection, changes in temperature, and even heightened emotion can produce the identical overreactive response of the body's cells.

How common are allergies?

Current estimates are that approximately 20 percent of all children will manifest some allergic symptoms at some time in their lives. From my experience I would say that this is an accurate estimate.

Can emotional upset cause allergy?

Anxiety in the child can indeed produce allergic symptoms since emotion is one of the basic triggers of the hyperreactive cell, just as allergy is. Emotion does not cause allergies, but can produce the identical symptoms and in addition can aggravate the symptoms produced by an allergic response.

What does it mean when the doctor says that he is an allergic child?

It means that he has demonstrated some allergic symptoms such as asthma, hay fever, and the like.

What is infectious allergy?

Infectious allergy occurs when the body responds to infection with a production of allergic symptoms. In children the most frequent example we see is the child who gets an ordinary cold but responds with wheezing and a deep, moist cough. In contrast, another child with the same viral cold may only have a slight stuffy nose and mild cough.

What about the child who has other allergies, not just "infectious allergy"?

This individual will always have the same allergy, but the body may react to it less as he gets older and therefore the symptoms may become milder.

Will he outgrow his allergies?

Yes, sometimes he will. For example, a child may only develop allergic symptoms in response to some sort of infection. If, for instance, he wheezes when he gets a cold and has no other signs of allergy he will gradually outgrow his problem, usually by four to five years of age. This is because the incidence of infection begins to decrease sharply around this time as the body builds up more and more immunity, and also because his bronchial tubes become larger, allowing more air to pass with less difficulty and therefore with less audible wheezing.

I realize that asthma and eczema are allergic disorders but what are some other symptoms of allergies in children? How do I know if my child is allergic?

Following are some symptoms which may result from allergy:

Listlessness and pallor.

Dark circles under the eyes.

Continual stuffy nose associated with the "allergic salute" —constant rubbing of the nose.

Persistent cough and congestion.

Frequent nosebleeds.

Recurrent abdominal pain.

Recurrent headaches.

The so-called tension fatigue syndrome, in which the child is listless, irritable, and always seems to look and feel below par.

In my experience many symptoms are often passed off as being emotional in origin that, in fact, have an allergic basis. Allergy is far more widespread than most people, physicians included, realize.

What is the most frequent cause of allergy in the environment?

In children dust is the number one offender. A good dust prevention routine, which your doctor can go over with you, can be invaluable in helping to rid your child as well as yourself of many unpleasant symptoms, such as runny nose, nighttime cough, etc.

Is air pollution a significant factor in producing allergic symptoms?

It definitely is. We see a great deal of eye irritation as well as nasal congestion when air quality deteriorates. Whether or not it leads to an increase in the incidence of infection is not yet established, but we do know that the combination of air pollution and high humidity is particularly bothersome in producing allergic symptoms.

Can little babies have allergies?

Yes, certainly. Allergies can make themselves known in the very first days of life. Some symptoms in infants include nasal stuffiness, vomiting and/or diarrhea, skin rashes, "colic," frequent spitting up, lots of "colds," and occasionally even wheezing.

What can I do to prevent allergies?

Reducing exposure to various allergens such as house dust and molds, to name two of the most important, will be of help if your child is allergic. Prolonged exposure to an allergen may cause him to develop an allergy to it even though he might tolerate it for a long period of time without symptoms.

Can you give me some guidelines to "allergy-proofing" my child's room?

Avoid upholstered furnishings and use simple designs in furniture that make it easier to clean and less likely to accumulate dust.

Keep closet doors closed and make sure that clothes are kept in the closet and not lying around the room. Wool clothes should be enclosed in plastic bags.

No fabric upholstery.

No rugs on the floor.

Allergy-proof casings for pillows, mattresses, and springs.

Paint walls or use a washable wallpaper, no pictures or other dust catchers.

Washable cotton or synthetic blankets, cotton bedspread.

No venetian blinds, just plain cotton or synthetic window-shades.

Cotton or fiber glass curtains, no draperies.

Window unit or central air conditioning so that windows may be kept closed at all times. No electric fans.

Synthetic materials for pillows.

Electric heater rather than hot-air duct heating. If you have the latter consider an electrostatic air filter or place cheesecloth over the vent in order to catch the dust and remember to change frequently.

Where are molds found?

"Mildew" or mold can accumulate on cheese and bread, as you well know, but it also develops in any damp area—for example, the shower stall or basement.

Have you any suggestions for reducing exposure to molds?

Avoid heavy vegetation around the house, which makes for increased dampness and thus the growth of molds.

Avoid stored foods that may produce mold.

Try to keep the leaves raked as they will provide an excellent source for mold growth.

Keep boots and sneakers "aired."

Avoid indoor plants.

Check the bathroom, wash the tiles frequently, and clean those corners where dampness easily collects and encourages mold growth.

Paint basements and other very damp areas with mold-inhibiting paint.

Dehumidify the cellar.

Vent clothes dryer to the outside to help keep the cellar dry.

Dry clothing immediately after laundering.

Use mold sprays to coat damp areas after washing them carefully.

What do you think about air filters? Will they help to reduce allergic symptoms such as nasal stuffiness?

I am all for them. An electronic air filter is best; although it is not cheap it will pay for itself in the relief of symptoms. Besides, the IRS will even allow it as a medical deduction if your physician so certifies. When you connect the filter to your forced-air system it is a good idea to keep the blower on constantly rather than intermittently since it constantly circulates and therefore filters the air. Don't worry about burning out the motor. Most of today's electric motors seem to run better when left on than when set to turn off and on automatically, which causes much more wear and tear.

What foods are most likely to provoke allergic symptoms?

Milk is far and away the most common troublemaker. Milk allergy is far more widespread than many parents and a good many physicians realize and can be the cause of many symptoms that are attributed to lots of other causes.

Chocolate, citrus fruits, cereal grains such as wheat and corn, egg white, strawberries, tomatoes, seafood, and peanut butter are the other most commonly involved foods.

Is it true that the younger the child the more likely that food is the cause of his allergy?

In general this is true, particularly with children under one year of age. This is not to say, however, that the baby cannot manifest symptoms to dust, molds, and other inhalants.

Can allergies develop before the baby is born?

Yes, the baby can be sensitized *in utero* by means of an allergen crossing the placenta, providing his first encounter with this substance. For example, a food eaten by the mother can produce allergic symptoms. Most of the time this does not occur and it will take several encounters with the allergen during infancy in order for the allergic individual to become sensitized to it.

TESTING AND TREATING ALLERGIES

What is skin testing for allergies?

A minute amount of a specific substance, such as a pollen, is given into the skin. If the body is allergic, a local reaction characterized by redness, swelling, and itching is produced. There is some correlation between the strength of the reaction and the strength of the allergy. A positive skin test means that the individual is allergic, but it does not necessarily mean that this substance is the cause of his present allergic difficulties. A negative test pretty well rules out the substance being a significant factor in the child's allergic problem.

I have heard that a child must be at least three years old before any skin testing for allergy can be done. Is this true?

No, it's not. Skin testing, if indicated, may be carried out in infancy.

I have heard that skin testing for allergy is very painful and upsetting to the child. Is this true?

Nothing can be more emotionally traumatic than an asthmatic attack. We parents routinely subject the child to various blood tests, and even surgery, such as tonsillectomy, but are afraid of skin testing. In skilled hands one can do just about all the skin tests necessary in one to three minutes, and they are practically painless, so don't let your child suffer needlessly because of this misconception.

What are allergy shots?

They are aqueous (water) extracts of the materials to which the child is allergic. These particles are carefully cleaned of any other foreign material and put into a sterile water solution so they can be given by injection. By giving small amounts of material to which the child is allergic over a period of time, the body may become desensitized—that is to say, it will learn not to overreact and produce allergic symptoms when confronted with the same material in larger doses.

Will repeated doses of an antibiotic make my child allergic to it?

No, it will not. He will not become allergic unless he is born with the capacity to be so. In an allergic individual repeated doses of a substance to which he is allergic can produce increasingly severe reactions, but he must be allergic to it to begin with.

SPECIFIC ALLERGIES

What is asthma?

Asthma means difficulty in breathing out that produces a wheezing sound. It is a clinical diagnosis and does not imply the cause of the difficulty. Most frequently allergy is at the root of the problem but other causes, such as an aspirated foreign body (like a peanut that may lodge in the bronchial tubes), may produce wheezing. Thus "asthma" needs to be evaluated by your doctor.

What are hives?

Hives are red, blotchy welts of varying sizes that usually itch and are produced by an allergic reaction of the body. Most of the time they go away quickly (within 24 to 48 hours) but sometimes can remain for several weeks. Occasionally the cause can be identified, but most of the time the trigger of the reaction remains unknown. Common causes include antibiotics such as penicillin and foods such as tomatoes, citrus fruits, and strawberries. An antihistamine prescribed by your doctor will be of great help in making your child more comfortable since it combats the body's allergic response.

I'm allergic to penicillin. Is the baby likely to be?

Specific allergies are not inherited, only the tendency to be allergic.

I had asthma as a child and my husband has hay fever as well as several other allergies. What are the chances of our baby developing allergies?

The chances are 65 to 75 percent that your baby will develop allergic symptoms. Only a milk allergy as such might possibly be inherited, but the tendency to develop allergic symptoms is indeed genetically transmitted. If only one parent has allergies, the chances of the offspring developing them are reduced to the neighborhood of 30 to 35 percent.

My child has a possible allergy to penicillin, but my doctor is not sure. Are there any tests available to make sure?

Actually there are only a very small number of children who are really allergic to penicillin, and this diagnosis needs to be made with as much accuracy and care as possible. If your child develops a rash while taking penicillin it is a good idea to have your doctor look at it to determine if it is allergic in nature. If your child breaks out in red welts (hives) that itch, he has the classic rash of an allergic response. Drug rashes frequently occur on the palms of the hands and soles of the feet (as well as elsewhere) whereas many other types, such as those caused by viruses, do not. Most frequently the situation arises where the child is taking penicillin for an infection and develops a rash that may be either infectious in nature or possibly allergic. Skin testing for penicillin allergy can be performed, but unfortunately can't give all the answers. A positive test means that penicillin allergy does exist, but a negative test does not rule out the possibility that the individual is sensitive. It is important to remember, however, that in some life-threatening situations it is possible to give even the penicillin-sensitive individual the drug by means of a technique of rapid desensitization that must be carried out in the hospital under carefully controlled conditions.

My child has a severe allergy to penicillin. Is there any way I can warn doctors about this in case I am not around and he should need treatment?

You bet there is. Write to Medic-Alert, a nonprofit organization based in Turlock, California 95880, and they will send you a tag that he should wear at all times.

What is eczema?

It is a chronic skin condition characterized by dry, scaly patches which most frequently occur in the bend of the elbows and behind the knees, but can occur almost anywhere on the body. In some individuals the skin reacts in this hypersensitive manner for reasons that are not fully understood. Occasionally contact agents such as wool are implicated and at times foods may play a role. Topical cortisone creams are useful in controlling itching and in clearing patches that are particularly annoying. Generalized eczema calls for more drastic measures.

Is poison ivy contagious?

No, but you can contract it if some of the oleoresin that causes the problem rubs off from the affected person onto your skin. By the same process it can be spread to other parts of the body as well. Be sure to wash all affected areas with soap and water immediately after exposure.

My child seems to get poison ivy every year. Is there something I can do to prevent it?

There are poison ivy shots available which, although far from being 100 percent effective, can work wonders in some cases. They must be given well in advance of the poison ivy season. Check with your doctor.

Can a person be allergic to cold?

Yes, he certainly can. This is a so-called physical allergy, which can also exist to heat and sun as well. Sensitivity to heat and cold usually manifests itself by the development of hives or swelling of various parts of the body. Photosensitivity to sun requires the combination of some drug to which the child is sensitive plus sunlight.

He has dark circles under the eyes. Does this mean that he is allergic?

Not necessarily, but there is no doubt that these dark circles are frequently seen in children who have allergies.

My child constantly rubs his nose and it always seems to be running. What does this mean?

It may mean that he is demonstrating what we refer to as the "allergic salute"; I would suggest that you look into allergy as a probable cause.

What can I do to prevent bee stings?

Wear plain clothing; avoid flowered prints, for example. Avoid perfumes and other sweet-smelling substances. Wear clothing that covers most of the body. It is also helpful to keep play areas clear of food and soft drinks.

What about an ordinary bee sting, where you get some localized painful swelling? What's the best thing to do?

Remove the stinger with tweezers if it is still in the skin. Then, if you have a little household ammonia, there is nothing better to neutralize the toxins. If not, apply a cold compress.

Which bees are most likely to cause allergic reactions?

The honeybee and the yellow jacket.

My child was stung by a bee on the hand and in a few minutes his hand was swollen and red. Does this mean he is allergic to bees stings? If so, what should be done about it?

As a general rule we do not worry about local reactions to bee stings. For example, if the child is stung on the hand, a local reaction would include swelling of the entire hand. If the swelling extends beyond the next joint, you should be concerned. Thus in the aforementioned instance, if the swelling should extend beyond the wrist, this would be cause for alarm. If he were stung on the foot and the swelling involved an area beyond the ankle and proceeded up the leg, this would be cause for further evaluation. In addition to this principle any systemic—that is, generalized—symptoms are cause for alarm. These include nausea, vomiting, nasal stuffiness, difficulty in breathing, and hives on other parts of the body. Any of these systemic symptoms mean that the individual is indeed allergic and needs to be immediately evaluated. If a child seems to have more of a reaction on a subsequent sting than he did on his first encounter, this also is a cause for alarm.

My child gets large welts whenever he is bitten by a mosquito or gnat. Is there something I should do about this?

No, it is just an individual variation in reactivity and nothing need be done.

13

Nervous System

CONVULSIONS

What should I do if my child has a convulsion?

Most convulsions in children are associated with fever and are of very short duration, less than a minute or two, and are over before you can do much of anything. In general, it is wise to turn the child on his right side with the head slightly down and hold him gently so that he will not injure himself. Do not plunge him in a tub of cold water, jam a stick or spoon in his mouth, or wrap him in a wet sheet. If the convulsion lasts more than a few minutes you should call the ambulance or rescue squad or otherwise head directly to the hospital.

What are the types of convulsions that you see in children?

Grand mal—A generalized convulsion with shaking and stiffening. This is the type seen with high fever, for example.

Petit mal—A brief absence attack (momentary loss of consciousness) characterized by a blank stare and occasionally fluttering of the eyelids. This is the type that may be noticed by the teacher at school and can cause learning disability.

Minor motor seizures—These lie somewhere in between the two above.

Myoclonic seizures—These are lightninglike jerking spells which most frequently occur in infancy and are usually very serious.

Psychomotor seizures—These are not common in children. They are associated with some type of behavioral abnormalities and most children who have them usually have other types of seizures as well.

Why is it necessary for my child to take anticonvulsants?

Your doctor has prescribed them for two basic reasons. First, there is evidence that the better controlled (less frequent) the seizures are, the better the chance that he will eventually stop having them. Secondly, anticonvulsants definitely decrease the risk of his having a very severe seizure that could produce brain damage.

My child has been taking anticonvulsant medication. How long will it be necessary for him to continue on it? He has not had any trouble in over two years.

There is no single answer for this one. It depends on your child's individual situation but, in general, after four years of being seizure-free, medication can be safely discontinued.

Do children tend to outgrow having convulsions?

Yes, there is a tendency for all types of seizure problems in children to improve with age, so time is on your side.

My child has had two convulsions. Both have occurred without fever. Is this epilepsy?

To me the term *epilepsy* should be reserved for those individuals who have had frequent seizures (convulsions) over a long period of time. Most pediatric neurologists would use the term *convulsive disorder* for your child.

My child has had two febrile convulsions. Can you tell me something about this problem?

Febrile convulsions occur frequently in otherwise healthy children. The tendency, as with all seizures in childhood, is for him eventually to outgrow them. The peak incidence is from one to three, and most of the time children no longer have them after age six or seven. They are usually of brief duration and do not result in any brain damage. You will want to discuss their treatment with your pediatrician.

Because he has had a febrile convulsion, will he have epilepsy?

No. The majority of children who have a seizure with fever either never have another one or outgrow the tendency entirely and are perfectly normal in every respect.

I am afraid that my child will become addicted to the medicine he is taking for his convulsive disorder. Is there a high incidence of this?

There is no cause for concern on this point. There are numerous well-documented studies of large series of children who have been followed for years while taking various anticonvulsants and addiction has not been a problem when they are withdrawn.

OTHER DISEASES

What is cerebral palsy?

This term is used to describe a child with brain damage apparent from birth. It does not tell anything about the cause of the damage or its extent, or what areas of the brain are affected. It is therefore a very general term.

My child gets frequent headaches. Are they common in children and what are some of the causes?

Headaches are very common in children. Some of the causes include:

Tension.

Allergy—Food allergies can occasionally be at fault, particularly milk, and a trial elimination diet often is helpful.

Migraine—Usually there is a family history. The headaches can be quite severe and are almost always associated with nausea and frequently vomiting. They may last up to several hours.

Brain tumor and cerebral vascular abnormalities—These are very rare causes of headache and most frequently there are other symptoms as well as abnormalities to be found on the examination.

Temporomandibular joint syndrome—A recently described problem of malocclusion of the jaw that can produce chronic headaches.

What is Down's syndrome?

This is a term now used in place of mongolism, which is a genetically determined kind of mental retardation associated with an oriental appearance to the face. Down was the English physician who first described the condition.

What can you tell me about sleepwalking?

It occurs at all ages but usually in the older child. I think that overstimulation and chronic fatigue play a significant role, so try to eliminate these factors and reduce any other anxiety and you will usually cure the problem. I have not run into any situations where the child has actually injured himself; but I would advise use of a chain lock on the room until the passage of time eliminates the habit.

HEAD INJURIES

My child just fell and bumped his head. What should I do?

Fortunately, most falls that children take are usually of a short distance and do not result in any loss of consciousness. The child usually cries and is upset but calms down with reassurance. It is wise, however, to know what symptoms indicate a potentially serious problem. Parents should be familiar with the following signs of head injury:

Loss of consciousness or progressively increasing lethargy or sleepiness.

Vomiting—Many children will vomit within a short time following a head injury and subsequently feel fine. If the vomiting occurs more than once or if it comes on several hours later, it may have far more serious implications.

Inequality of the pupils—The dark spots in the eyes should be equal on both sides.

Crossing of the eyes and double vision.

Inability to move the arms equally well on both sides.

Mental clarity—He doesn't know who he is, who you are, etc.

Convulsion.

Stiff neck.

In addition to vomiting the child is also frequently sleepy. This may be because he has been so emotionally upset by the event that he is exhausted. It is all right to let him lie down and even sleep providing you rouse him at frequent intervals and make sure that none of the above danger signs is developing. I usually advise doing the same thing through the night, perhaps two or three times. Another point I have found helpful is to give him only a light meal if he is due for one, for anything more may prove nauseating.

With regard to the severity of head injury in addition to the above, memory of the event is an important criterion. In the younger child this may be difficult to assess, but essentially the longer the period of amnesia extends back before the injury, the more severe it is. This is known as *duration of retrograde amnesia.*

Should he have a skull X-ray?

This decision will be up to your doctor, of course. However, even if the skull X-ray is taken and does not reveal any fracture of the bone, a serious problem can still develop. So always watch for the signs of head injury—regardless of whether or not the skull X-ray has shown anything.

14

Safety

AVOIDING ACCIDENTS

Accidents remain by far the leading cause of death in children, and despite all the talk and magazine articles, we still see far too many easily preventable accidents in children. Here are some general safety tips which should prove helpful:

Never leave young children (under ten) alone in the house.

Never leave a young child alone in the bathroom or kitchen; these are the two most dangerous rooms in the house.

Always use the back burners on the stove and remember that more accidents occur in the kitchen than anywhere else in the house.

Use a gate for the stairs until he has shown he knows how to negotiate them.

Cover unused electrical outlets with plastic plug covers.

Don't leave the baby alone with a sibling under the age of eight and then only for a short period of time while you are elsewhere in the house.

Do not assume a child under four years of age will follow instructions. He will cross that busy street at the first opportunity.

Never leave an infant on a changing table or bed unattended. Even if he is supposedly unable to roll over he may well pick that instant to accomplish this feat for the first time. Furthermore, you will notice that even a newborn baby can really wiggle around, so be careful. Falls of this type continue to be far too common. Never take your hands off the baby! If you must reach down for something, always keep one hand firmly on him.

Use bumper guards for infants in the crib and make sure that the crib has slats that are closely spaced so that he cannot get caught in them.

Never give peanuts to a child under six years of age as he may easily swallow them, especially if it is at adult cocktail time and he is racing around excitedly.

Balloons can be dangerous for the child under four since they may lodge tightly in the back of the throat if accidentally swallowed.

Chewable vitamins can also be easily swallowed and cause choking in the young child. The chances are that his diet is well enough balanced and fortified so that he doesn't need them anyway.

Avoid tight-fitting clothing, especially infant stretch suits that can be very tight around the ankles and wrists.

Always throw out unused medicine.

Lock up medicine, solvents, etc.

Never keep anything in the house whose contents are not clearly labeled.

Don't rely on safety devices to keep a nonswimming child safe in the water.

Never pull or swing your child by his outstretched arms as this can dislocate the arm. It is wise that parents be instructed in reducing a dislocation of the arm themselves, as it may occur in a place where medical attention is not available. I am amazed at how few physicians know how to do it, so ask your pediatrician to demonstrate it and learn what a simple and painless procedure it is.

Be extremely cautious about taking the infant out in the direct sun. Remember he will show no signs of difficulty until after he has been burned, so you must remember to shield him carefully. Expose him to approximately three to five minutes of direct sunlight and judge how much skin reaction this induces. Build up gradually from this point unless the child is very fair-skinned or a redhead or unless there is a strong family history of skin cancer, in which case it may be wise to use some sort of sun screen.

If all is quiet and the children are not in sight, go and see what he or they are up to, for chances are they are up to no good!

Never leave a child alone in the bathtub until you are sure he is old enough to handle himself if he should slip underwater.

Never use a pillow in the crib or bassinet while the baby (under six months) is sleeping.

Never keep plastic bags around the house. Children can and have suffocated from becoming entrapped in them.

Beware of rope and cord used while climbing trees or on the swing.

Make sure if you use a pacifier that it is safe and will not come apart, nor is made in such a way that it can accidentally lodge in the back of the throat and cause choking and possibly suffocation.

Beware of your child eating any plant. There are many that you may have in your garden or house that are highly toxic, such as oleander, philodendron, privet, buttercup, wisteria, yew, and yellow jasmine, to mention a few.

Make it a general rule to train your child *never* to put any plant in his mouth.

Accidents are more likely to occur when there is some increased level of stress in the home—illness, moving, fatigue, emotional discord, etc. So at these times be doubly careful.

Coffee tables with sharp edges are a safety hazard and produce numerous cuts and bruises of the head and scalp.

Keep the local poison control number handy.

Know your nearest emergency room facility, where it is located, and how to get there.

Automobile safety—Infants and children up to age four years or 40 inches should not use standard seat belts as they can cause abdominal trauma. Infant and young child (age one to five) carriers are available such as the GM model. Children over four years may use seat belts and those older (four and a half feet in height) may use the shoulder harness.

According to the Committee on Accident Prevention of the American Academy of Pediatrics there were 5796 deaths from automobile accidents in 1973 in children 14 years of age and under.

Most important, know your child. There are some who are born curious and will remain so for the rest of their lives. There are some who are definitely accident-prone. If you have one of these you will have to be extra cautious. The same is true for the child who is fearless, a tendency that can be spotted in early infancy. He will be the one who jumps into the pool when your back is turned or winds up on the high diving board when he is only two. Face it—these types demand more careful supervision.

If your child has ingested anything he shouldn't, remember the odds are strongly in favor of his repeating the performance. Recognition of your child's particular personality pattern early can be the single most important factor in preventing a serious accident later on.

Do not let a young child draw his own tap water for a bath. There have been cases where the water drawn from the tap was hot enough to scald the skin.

Beware of the danger of the second cup of coffee in the morning. Just as you have gotten the eldest fed and off to school in the car pool and you sit down to read the morning paper with your nice hot cup of coffee, along comes your toddler, who reaches up and pulls it off.

Make sure you educate your child regarding matches and do not leave them around where they are easily accessible to young children.

Be extremely cautious about the use of extension cords for various appliances that may then be unplugged. Children frequently pick up the cord and chew on the end. This can cause a very serious electrical burn of the face and mouth.

Be extremely careful not to leave an infant or young child in the car with the windows rolled up in hot weather. No doubt you have heard this advice in regard to the family pet but don't forget the same thing applies to children as well.

15

Emotional Matters

DISCIPLINE

How should I discipline him? Should I spank him?

I think it depends on the offense, the age, and your own personal feelings in the matter. To my way of thinking, for a major offense endangering himself or others—playing with matches, turning on the stove, crossing the street unattended, etc.—I think the punishment should be a stiff one and therefore use of the hand or hairbrush on the rear end is not out of order. I do not care for physical discipline as a rule and reserve it essentially for these occasions. Hand patting, wrist slapping, and the like are for the birds; better no tap at all than a meaningless one. The basis of good discipline is to teach, not to punish, so remember always to make clear to your child at any age exactly what you are disciplining him for. The method will vary greatly from one family to another, but use the one most effective in getting your point across. If you are going to mete out punishment make sure that it is done as close to the event as possible, particularly when dealing with the young child, who quickly forgets what he has done. If you find yourself needing to discipline your child frequently you had better take time to look over the whole situation and ask why. Also make sure the child knows what behavior you expect from him and what the consequences of not behaving in this fashion will be. Be sure you teach him in advance so that he knows where you stand. This is a good way to avoid the necessity for frequent discipline.

My six-year-old's behavior has recently become extremely negative. He repeatedly disobeys and is willful. How should I handle it?

The recent development of undesirable behavior should make you look carefully in the environment, family, school, or neighborhood for the cause. Has there been a separation at home—a move, for example? There is always some explanation for a child's behavior, and although it may not be readily apparent, it can and must be found. The worst thing to do is to fall into the trap of chasing the symptoms without taking the time to find the cause. If you can't come up with a satisfactory answer, seek professional help by starting with your pediatrician.

My five-year-old asked me if he could do something the other day and even though I couldn't think of any good reason why not I just felt that I should say no. Now I feel guilty about it. Should one always have a logical reason?

In theory, yes, though many times your gut reaction is to say no. Let your conscience be your guide; trust yourself. Chances are you would not feel that way unless there was a good reason, even though you can't put your finger on it at the time. Stick to your guns and as long as you feel that you are doing your best, it will all come out all right.

I have to ask him two or three times to do everything. How do I get him to pay attention?

To begin with, I don't know of any parent who hasn't had this problem. Now, ask yourself whether any of the following applies to you:

1. Are you asking him to do too much?
2. Are you probably asking him too frequently?
3. Do you follow through, or do you give up in exasperation after the third or fourth time?
4. Do you waver between the "I give up" and the volcanic explosion with hairbrush in hand, with the result that he never knows which extreme to expect?
5. Do you threaten him with a multitude of punishments, but never follow through with any of them?
6. Have you become much more oriented in the direction

of thinking about what disciplinary measure to use next and have you forgotten to praise him in any positive way on those seemingly rare occasions when he does what you ask?

If one or more of these are true, then it is time to regroup and begin again. Start by sitting down with him (it is best if both parents are involved) and go over a few (one to three) things you will expect and why. Be consistent (parental agreement beforehand), brief, reasonable, and honest. Let him also know the consequences of not performing. If he is to be punished, he should know in advance for what and how. Finally, and most important, you must follow through with what you have told him. Be true to your words or he will feel you have let him down, as indeed you have. This is just as true with regard to a punishment as with a promise to take him to the football game.

Gradually, as he gets older, you can add more responsibility; in fact, he will expect more as recognition of his increased maturity.

New Arrivals

When shall I tell him he is adopted?

I would begin to use the term early on, before you are even sure he understands, so that the word itself becomes familiar to him. By age three he will begin to take in some of its significance and may even find the term used in a peer group. By five years of age he is ready for some explanation and you should give him one as truthful and as simplified as possible. If you obtained him through a reputable adoption agency then you can tell him that it was quite a process all three of you went through to assure everyone concerned that you were meant for each other. Don't go overboard and launch into a detailed account, which often only serves to communicate your insecurity about telling him. Your naturalness in handling the situation will do more to allay his anxieties than any other single factor.

How about spacing the family? When is the best time to have another child?

When you feel you want another child, it's time to go ahead. There's no ideal time as far as I am concerned. The closer siblings are in age the more intense the rivalry, but this has no bearing on the individual situation. Of course, the sex of the new arrival has a bearing on this, but I think that the overriding factor is the parents' positive feelings about adding to the family. Let *your* instincts guide you and not the latest article in this month's magazine.

When should I tell my two-year-old that a baby is on the way?

It continues to fascinate me that children seem to know at the same time you do that you are pregnant. It is never too early to tell them that the baby is on the way. Now obviously one doesn't have to go into great detail, when it's still some months away, but it is certainly no secret!

Divorce and Separation

My husband and I are separated. Will this affect my child?

It certainly will, so be prepared for some adjustment problems. Even an infant is likely to show some form of behavioral difficulty, such as increased fussiness, poor sleep patterns, and the like. The toddler will frequently become more "clingy" and the older child may become defiant and openly hostile. The best way to understand the effects of separation on the child is to think of it from his point of view. He will find the event almost impossible to understand and very frightening. If his parents can suddenly part ways, then they can just as suddenly abandon him altogether. You can allay a great deal of his anxiety by preparing him well in advance. State, for instance, that the two of you don't get along well living together and you have decided to live apart for a while to see if it will improve the situation. Assure him that you both still love him and that you do not contemplate leaving him, that you both remain just as interested as ever in his welfare. Talk to him about it and let him talk to you. Even if there is a great deal of discord and bitterness between the two of you, try to cool it when it comes to the children since the separation itself is traumatic enough in their eyes.

How will divorce affect the children?

Usually I find that a final settlement of your affairs and putting your house in order again has a much more positive effect on the child than you anticipated. He will feel much more secure once he knows what the situation is, and as you become more stabilized, so will he. The final resolution of your situation through a divorce is usually much easier for a child to accept than is a separation. In today's world it is such a frequent event that he will certainly be exposed to peers who have been through the same thing. There is just no avoiding causing the children emotional suffering during the uncoupling process. On the other hand, they might well have suffered far more remaining in a home full of discord or a basic lack of compatibility. The situation will not be insurmountable, and may well open a much happier phase of your life. Make sure you communicate this attitude to the children.

SPEECH PROBLEMS

He talks baby talk.

This is particularly true of the preschooler with a younger sibling. He figures that the more he acts like the youngest member of the family, the more attention he will get. Your actions in making sure that he feels secure about his place in the family will allay this anxiety and go a long way toward combatting the natural tendency toward regressive behavior. Such regressive baby talk is to be distinguished from difficulty with consonant sounds, which may persist up to age six or seven. Seldom does this type of speech need any therapy and it almost always self-corrects with time.

My child is four years old and at times seems to speak immaturely. His teacher says that he might need speech therapy. What do you think?

Immature speech is what I call a functional problem and usually is self-correcting if you give it time. If his peers seem to understand him, chances are that he does not have a serious problem and probably doesn't need any therapy.

He stutters. What shall I do?

All children go through a normal phase of stuttering at about three years of age in which syllables or words are repeated. Your approach should be to *ignore it entirely*—educated neglect, I like to call it. Do not ask him to repeat the word or tell him that if he tries hard he can do it better. If he begins to feel you are concerned he will become more and more anxious, which will only serve to make matters worse. Be sure to give him ample time to express himself and to listen carefully to what he has to say so that he does not feel under pressure to get it all out quickly before his audience disappears. If your child continues to stutter and is still doing so by age four he will need careful management. This condition is far more common in boys, for reasons that are not understood. There is no magic cure, but all people who deal with the problem are convinced that no direct attention should be focused on it, but rather on an examination of the environment for avoidable causes of stress.

DEALING WITH DEATH

My wife recently died of cancer. My 12-year-old son doesn't seem to be too upset now that the initial shock has passed, but he is quieter and less communicative and seems to have trouble sleeping at night. What should I do?

This is an instance, although fortunately rare in pediatric practice, that demands expert guidance. The loss of a parent can have catastrophic effects on the child, and even though little disturbance may be apparent on the surface, a great deal is going on in his mind. Communication is of the essence, and it should be with a trained expert, such as a child psychiatrist, and not an amateur who may do more harm than good. Even a younger child who has lost a parent deserves the opportunity to talk it out with such a person.

His grandfather died of cancer. What shall I tell him?

The answer is, of course, dependent on the age of your child. The principles, however, are the same at all ages. First, make sure you do talk to him about it. Be honest and avoid making up some pleasant-sounding explanation since he will find out the truth sooner or later. Be brief, but take time to answer all of his questions in the same straightforward manner. He will lose the point if the discussion is too drawn out. Also, I think it is wise to bring the subject up occasionally to make sure there are no unanswered questions or misunderstandings. It is crucial to remember that his attitude about death and his way of handling and accepting it will depend on how you react more than anything else.

His grandfather died. Should I take him to the funeral?

There are two factors here: the age of the child and the closeness of the relationship between the child and the deceased. Generally speaking, if the relationship was close and the child is over three years old I think that it is acceptable and even a good idea that he attend the funeral. You will have to be supportive and answer the inevitable questions. Where there will be a "viewing" I would hesitate to take a child under 12.

STEALING

Yesterday I found a toy car in his room that I know does not belong to him. How shall I handle it?

First of all recognize that all children will take something that is not theirs at some point in their lives, so don't overreact! Be straightforward and ask him about it, explaining that even though it does not belong to him, you will not punish him if he is truthful and tells you where he got it. You are trying to keep the channels of communication open at all times, so don't descend on him in a threatening manner. Once you have started the dialogue explain why it is not a good idea to take from others. Be forthright, but gentle. Remember, he already feels bad enough about it to begin with and compounding his guilt will only make him more reluctant to tell about similar transgressions in the future. Do not go back on your word and punish him after you have stated that you would not. You should probably have him return the toy, but in certain situations this may prove too much of an embarrassment to him, and you may compound difficulties by forcing him. In these instances you might have to do it for him. Keep in mind that you are trying to get across the point that if he tells you about his misdeeds, not only will he be assured that you will not unjustly punish him, but he will feel much better in being able to communicate.

What about repeated stealing?

For the most part this represents an acting-out process on the part of the child by which he fulfills some unmet needs. He is usually insecure and feels threatened and it is your job as a parent to try to figure out why. Don't immediately blame yourself and don't just mete out one punishment after another, but step back and try to look at the situation from his point of view. Is he being outdone by his siblings? Is school going badly? Have you been forced to travel a lot recently and not been able to spend time with him? Is there marital discord? These are but a few of the reasons why a child can feel insecure. Attacking the problem in this manner may lead to a constructive solution, but repetitive discipline, which often grows harsher and harsher, will have no beneficial effect. Most of the time those objects that are taken are never used, but only secreted away, and some are even placed so as to be "found." There is therefore a need that is not being met and a desire to call this to your attention. React accordingly!

LEAVING HIM WITH OTHERS

Any suggestions on selecting a housekeeper? Both my husband and I will be working full time.

I prefer someone of the same cultural background, if possible. Certainly it should be a person who loves children and can effectively work with them. To heck with the messy house as long as the children are happy and well cared for. Look for someone who agrees with your general philosophy of child rearing. Avoid the dominant type who tries to replace you in the eyes of your child. It is a big responsibility to select someone who will participate to such a large extent in shaping your children, particularly those in the preschool age group. Give it plenty of time and thought and make sure you have a trial period to observe the interaction between your housekeeper and your children. Finally, select someone you feel is basically a person who cares.

We are planning a trip to Europe for two weeks. What should I tell my child?

Of course the content depends on the age, but the principle is the same. For the preschooler, tell him a week or two in advance. By that time he will have already figured it out since you will have been rushing around long before that getting ready! Be truthful, direct, and succinct. No long-winded explanations or descriptions, and you don't need to justify your actions, unless of course this is your fourth trip abroad this year! Don't feel guilty you are doing it, but instead go ahead and enjoy your trip. If he feels you are happy about it, he will feel secure as well.

SCHOOL RESISTANCE

My child complains of stomachaches or headaches in the morning and says he does not feel well enough to go to school. The doctor has checked him out and says there's is nothing wrong. What shall I do?

An occasional demonstration of the Monday morning blues is quite normal and universal, and I would urge you to tell him that even though he might not feel up to par he will feel better once he gets up and gets going. Don't belittle his symptoms or tell him he is just making them up, but don't give in either! If this pattern continues, it's time to search out the cause. There is something going on that he has felt unable or unwilling to communicate or perhaps that he doesn't recognize himself. He needs help, so don't hesitate to seek advice.

My five-year-old screams bloody murder when the car pool arrives to take him to school. I've tried to take him myself but it doesn't do any good. How shall I handle it?

First of all recognize that it is a common problem and this separation anxiety is usually short-lived. Play it cool, be firm and consistent, and, above all, don't give in! The less reaction you show the more secure your child will feel about leaving you. If, on the other hand, you become anxious and indecisive, he will say, "I'm right. She is as concerned as I am about my leaving home."

My child seems to be having trouble getting to sleep at night. I think he is worrying about school. I wonder about giving him some medication to help him sleep. What do you think?

I am amazed at the number of times I am asked to prescribe some sort of sedation for children. With rare exceptions, I am totally opposed to giving out any sedatives in pediatric practice. Teaching reliance on a pill of one sort or another cannot help but lead to difficulty later on and may well predispose your child to being a chronic pill taker for the rest of his life. It is a far better policy to spend the time and effort trying to understand and solve his problems than to take the easy way out and treat the symptoms but let the real problem go unattended. You and he will both benefit greatly by learning to work through the anxiety, live with some degree of frustration, and then develop a solution.

MISCELLANEOUS

He bites his nails.

An age-old habit for which there is still no magic solution. It is a symptom of tension and therefore you should look for any stressful conditions that might easily be eliminated or at least eased. Foul-tasting preparations applied to the fingernails offer no help and usually the more one reprimands the worse the situation becomes, although an occasional brief discussion of what an unattractive habit it is may prove helpful. I have also had considerable success by having the child look in the mirror while performing his nail-biting routine. Seeing how really unattractive it looks may be enough to cause its demise.

My four-year-old wakes up at night screaming. What shall I do?

There are two basic kinds of frightening nocturnal events. One is the nightmare and the other the night terror. With nightmare the child awakens crying but is awake and able to communicate when you arrive. He is frequently scared out of his wits and needs brief reassurance that none of what took place was real. In the other situation the child partially awakens screaming but is really not fully in touch when you attempt to communicate with him and may never really awaken, but with gentle holding and soothing conversation will usually go back to sleep. Both of these occur because of active dream states and in my experience are associated with fatigue and overstimulation. Instituting regular naps for the preschooler as well as a decent bedtime hour for all ages and avoiding overuse of the "tube" will go a long way toward decreasing the level of stimulation and often seems to eliminate the problem.

My five-year-old is afraid of the dark. Do you approve of leaving a light on?

I certainly do, and well remember being in the same boat myself.

My seven-year-old is a "middle child." Do you think there is such a thing as the "middle child" syndrome?

Yes, I think that many children, be they middle children or not, at times feel pressure from above or below or both in the pecking order. Most of the time they will respond well to some individual attention by one or both parents. Make sure you make some time available and be sure to listen carefully during these periods and you will gain a great deal more insight into your child.

He uses a lot of bad words. I'm amazed. How shall I handle it?

Children usually begin to throw out a few choice four-letter blockbusters at about five, sometimes even earlier. They have heard them from their peers, and occasionally even at home. They don't know what they mean but have quickly learned that they have great shock value. Their use is based entirely on seeing the reaction they produce. So, meet the situation head on but don't gasp and throw up your arms. Merely state in a straightforward manner that such language is not acceptable because it can offend or hurt other people. You might add that you have heard these words before and there's nothing new about his recent discovery. Usually that's enough, for you have successfully taken the wind out of his sails without giving him the idea that you are bristling and ready to do instant battle. If he persists in dropping these choice little numbers, he deserves punishment, but this is usually not necessary.

My ten-year-old frequently complains of abdominal pain. Do you think he could have an ulcer?

Recurrent abdominal pain is a frequent symptom in children and needs evaluation by a doctor. An ulcer is a rare cause but other more common causes include tension, urinary-tract infections, allergy, and constipation.

My five-year-old walked into our bedroom the other night while we were having intercourse. He didn't seem nearly as shook up as we were, but what should I tell him?

I would tell him a couple of things. First of all, when a door is closed you don't open it without announcing yourself with a call or a knock. This is a good rule to follow on any occasion. I would then explain to him that you and his father (or mother, depending on who is doing the talking) love each other very much and to show your affection you sometimes hug and kiss vigorously when you are in bed. You do not need to launch into a detailed explanation but make sure that you discuss it with him since the confrontation is usually far more upsetting to the child than to you. Remember, he doesn't know what you were doing.

I have read a lot about sibling rivalry, but in this case it is my older child who seems to be having the problems. Is this unusual?

Certainly not. Most of the time we think of the younger child as having to adjust to big brother, but often the younger one is becoming a holy terror and the oldest ends up taking it on the chin. Since he is older, bigger and, we hope, wiser, more is to be expected of him. Still, don't expect too much. If his behavior has suddenly become difficult, it may be that you need to set more limits on the younger member or members of the group!

My daughter seems to have a great deal of discomfort with her periods. What can I do to help her?

In my experience many of the symptoms of discomfort with menstrual periods are emotional in origin. It's important to reassure adolescent girls that this is a frequent complaint, does not mean anything is wrong with them, will not occur with every period for the rest of their lives, and that anxiety and emotional tension can aggravate and occasionally precipitate the problem. If the attitude about menstruation has been a healthy, positive one, the incidence of this difficulty will be far less later on, so make sure your young lady is properly informed in a positive and supportive manner.

What we try hard to avoid is giving out lots of medication for symptoms associated with periods since I am firmly convinced that this can and does lead to dependency on first one kind of medication and then another. Occasional aspirin, relieving tension where possible, and encouraging your daughter to remain active during her period will all work toward lessening the problem and, in many cases, cure it entirely.

My child was sexually molested. She is seven years old and refuses to tell me anything more specific than that she was approached and touched by a stranger. What should I do?

You will want to talk with your pediatrician. In virtually all cases of child molestation I think that referral to a child psychiatrist is indicated. It is of the utmost importance that the child be allowed to communicate feelings about the incident, which is best done to a trained listener who can help the child interpret the events in a realistic and helpful manner. Usually a few sessions on a short-term basis is enough to restore a feeling of normalcy to the child as well as the parents.

He just won't eat. What should I do?

This question ranks well up in the top ten! Most often it is asked about the one-year-old whose appetite drops off and for good reason. His growth rate drops off rather precipitously at this age. But regardless of the child's age my answer is nearly always the same. "Don't worry." Several excellent studies have conclusively shown that given the opportunity to eat a balanced diet a child will select one himself. It is only when we parents get ourselves into the act that we get in so much hot water. For the year-old child you should put out a balanced meal and then turn your back, not in a literal sense necessarily, but at least emotionally. If he gets the idea that you are waiting with bated breath to see what he eats, he will quickly begin to use what and how much as a weapon. Sure, he'll occasionally knock most of it on the floor, and there will often be times when you will feel a total failure, convinced that he will starve to death and you better get another pediatrician. But if he doesn't eat at one meal, he will make it up at another. No otherwise healthy young child is going to stop eating to the point where he will put himself in any nutritional jeopardy, but many will give you fits. So don't get into a pitched battle with him, and tell the grandparents to relax as well. Under no circumstances should you begin to offer food if he acts hungry after mealtime. This will quickly begin a vicious cycle where he is always hungry and you are feeding him throughout the day. When this happens, it's the attention he wants and he is smart enough to eat only a small amount so he will be the center of attention again an hour later. Once you pack things up after a sufficient length of time, say an hour at most, that's it. He will catch on fast. By handling mealtimes and food in this way you will avoid attaching more emotional significance to the amount and kind of food your child eats than is healthy for him.

16

Education

What about all these cognitive toys? Do you think they aid in development?

No. Most children I see have an environment that is already sufficiently enriched to provide all the ingredients for intellectual growth. Contrived manipulation of your child in order to make him smarter will only rob him of the enjoyment of learning spontaneously under guidance that is not always goal-directed. Do what comes naturally.

My six-year-old reverses a lot of his letters and even writes whole words backwards. Should I be concerned?

A great many children in the five- to seven-year-old age group will demonstrate so-called mirror writing. The vast majority of them pass through this stage spontaneously. This is a normal stage of development and you should make no attempt to correct the child.

SCHOOLING

What type of preschool do you think is best?

I prefer a low-keyed school situation which, although possessing some structure, is not rigid in its format. You will want to visit around yourself; be sure to start well ahead of time since the great demand for preschool education means the better ones fill early.

What about open classrooms? Are you in favor of them?

It is extremely difficult for most children to maintain the self-discipline required in an open classroom situation. The self-motivation required in such a setting is also unusual for children, particularly in the early grades. For a few exceptionally bright and motivated individuals the open classroom is undoubtedly successful, but for the majority of children I think it is disastrous.

My son has a birthday in November. Do you think he should wait a year before starting the first grade?

This is a difficult question to answer with a general statement, but I would say that, as a rule, having a boy with a late birthday spend an extra year at the preschool level is often a fine idea. The same may also be true with a girl, although girls have less in the way of learning problems in the primary years. Too often a child who is one of the youngest in the class must constantly struggle to keep up. The result is frequently anxiety and unhappiness. The longer the situation has been allowed to go on, the more difficult it is even to consider repeating a grade since the child's self-image may be damaged. All this means is that you should think it over carefully before he enters the first grade and make your decision while he is still at the preschool level.

Are you in favor of public or private schools?

Parents frequently seem to ask pediatricians for educational advice although we are not educators. Since we have known your child since birth, this makes good sense. I feel quite strongly that a school should be selected on the basis of your individual child. You should seek an environment that will enable him to achieve his potential and your and his expectations. Furthermore, it should provide an educational atmosphere where your child will be happy and well adjusted. For some this is a small private school with a rigid curriculum while for others it is a large class in the public school system. Far too often, in my experience, parents select the school first and think of their child second; it should be the other way around. You should also bear in mind that education today is a long haul and may not mean only college, but graduate school as well. The child who is emotionally well adjusted to his school environment in the early and formative years is far more likely to pursue his education when the choice to do so becomes his own.

Do you think it is important that a school offer "frill" courses such as music and art?

I think it is of great importance. Far more emphasis should be placed in these areas, as they are most important avenues toward the development of the child's innate creativity.

My child seems to be having difficulty with his homework. I have tried to help him, but it only seems to make matters worse. What do you suggest?

Instead of tackling his homework I would try to look for the reason why he is having trouble completing it. Is the work too difficult for him? Is there difficulty at school with peers or with the teacher? Is there some recent situation that has produced emotional tension? As a general rule, helping with homework to some extent is certainly acceptable, but when it becomes a routine requirement and is developing into teaching on a regular basis one should be concerned. More often than not a serious problem needs to be uncovered and intelligently dealt with, the earlier the better. It is neither necessary nor desirable to have parents take over the role of teacher.

How do I know if he is doing well in school?

If he gets up on his own in the morning, dresses, and comes bouncing downstairs for breakfast while you're still half asleep, then the odds are overwhelming that everything at school is A-OK!

Will eye exercises help him to read?

I don't think so. After all, reading is a central brain function and has nothing to do with the eyes themselves. Despite what you may have read, there is no good evidence that exercising the eyes will make the brain function better.

I am taking my child to the pediatrician because of school difficulties. What can I do to make the visit of maximum benefit and what can I expect?

You can help by sending in all pertinent information well ahead of time—for example, a report from the school, previous medical records, results of any previous intellectual testing, and the like. I stress "well ahead of time" so your doctor can go over these reports. You can count on at least two visits since your child will need a complete physical examination if he has not had one recently and your pediatrician will want to do some screening of his learning abilities. In addition, he will take the history of the problem and will want to sit down and talk with both parents if possible. As you can see, this cannot be done in the midst of a busy day and needs some special scheduling. Your pediatrician will probably refer your child for some sort of psychometric (IQ-type testing) by a psychologist and may order other tests he thinks necessary.

LEARNING DISABILITIES

The teacher says he has learning problems and that he should have a neurological examination and may need a brain-wave test as well. What would you suggest?

I would suggest strongly resisting any tendency to panic. Just slow down and don't let the teacher or school stampede you. Call your pediatrician and talk it over with him and follow his guidance as to how to proceed further. This may mean making an appointment to sit down in the office (both parents) and discuss fully what the problem seems to be from the school's and parents' point of view. In my experience this often leads to a relatively straightforward solution, and it may not even be necessary to go off to the neurologist, psychiatrist, or psychologist to perform a host of unnecessary tests. This is not to be construed as advice to make light of or to disregard the school's diagnosis of a learning problem.

What about an EEG?

An EEG, or eclectroencephalogram (brain-wave test), is not necessary in the routine evaluation of a child with a learning problem. If there is a history of convulsions, momentary lapses of consciousness, or suspicion of some other neurological abnormality, your doctor may order an EEG as well as other studies.

What about psychological testing? The school mentioned that this might be helpful in evaluating his learning problem.

I think that a good psychological evaluation done by someone who works a great deal with children is the single most important method of evaluating the child with a learning problem. A good psychologist will not only be able to evaluate the child's intellectual capabilities, but also will be able to give the parents as well as the physician insight into his emotional situation.

How do I go about arranging for a psychological test?

You can either have this evaluation done through the school system or privately. If you choose the latter route it is best to ask your pediatrician for a recommendation. Make sure that the results of the evaluation are forwarded to him.

Just what does this psychological evaluation consist of?

The psychologist will first take a history of your child's learning difficulty and gather information about your family in general. Next, your child will be given various standardized tests, and scores for each will be computed. These tests cover various areas of brain function such as mathematical ability, memory, and verbal performance, from which may be determined a general level of intellectual function (IQ). But it is just as important to obtain an idea of how your child performs in each specific area. For example, he may score very well in tests requiring mathematical skills and yet do poorly in those requiring him to read. This discrepancy in abilities, despite an overall normal level of function computed by averaging the different subtest scores, may be at the root of his learning problem. An evaluation of the child's emotional status is every bit as important as his intellectual performance. This may include formal testing, such as the Rorschach or other methods, and general conversation with a skilled professional.

What can be done for the child with a learning disability?

Most important is to make the correct diagnosis. This consists of trying to determine what is the root cause of the difficulty. Is it the so-called minimal brain dysfunction syndrome or is it a primary emotional problem? Perhaps chronic untreated allergy is at the bottom of it or a difficulty with hearing or an unrecognized seizure problem. There are many possible causes and your pediatrician is the one who will work with you in arriving at the proper diagnosis.

The second most important factor in helping your child is to understand the nature of his learning problem and what causes it. After a thorough diagnostic evaluation, which your doctor will help you plan, those involved should sit down with you and discuss their findings in detail until you feel that you have grasped your child's difficulty.

If he does indeed have an organic learning disability, specific educational planning is of prime importance and this, of course, is the responsibility of the educator. I do feel, however, that the pediatrician should be involved in this process, as it is he who has the best overall picture of the total child. Educational planning may result in the placement of your child in a special learning disabilities class, arrangements for remedial tutoring, perhaps a change in school, or some other suggestions.

What is the incidence of learning disabilities in children?

Estimates vary from 8 to as high as 15 percent of the population.

Are there other terms used to denote learning problems?

Yes, there are a good many. Included are:

Dyslexia—This term originally referred to certain people who had extreme difficulty with reading and applied exclusively to this difficulty with the written word, but now it is used interchangeably with other terms to denote a learning disability. It is certainly true that most children with minimal brain dysfunction have difficulty with reading but this is not always the case.

Minimal brain damage—This term is frequently used but

in my opinion incorrectly. It implies that there has been some sort of brain damage that has taken place and is responsible for the child's learning problem. But the vast majority of these children have *no* evidence whatsoever of *any* sort of brain damage. To label a child in this manner is irresponsible in my opinion and can lead to considerable psychological harm. In a small number of children there may indeed have been some organic injury to the brain that has produced brain damage, but this group accounts for only a small percentage of the total number of children with learning problems and this term should be applied only to this group, if used at all.

Special learning disability—Special classes for these children are often referred to as SLD classes or programs.

Hyperactive child—Children with learning disabilities are frequently hyperactive but such is not always the case. Furthermore a child may be hyperactive and yet have no learning problems.

The terms " organic learning disability," "exceptional child," and "special child" are also used to refer to the learning-disabled child.

What does the term MBD mean? I seem to see it every time I pick up a magazine.

MBD stands for minimal brain dysfunction. It is a term that is applied to a wide range of learning problems and is not a specific diagnosis. What is usually meant is a child who has an overall normal IQ, but who has marked irregularities in his performance. For example, he may be very good with mathematical skills, but do very poorly in those areas which require verbal abilities. His overall score in a series of tests, when averaged out, is solidly in the normal range, but of course this does not tell the story since he will have great difficulties performing in his weak areas. In the majority of children designated as having MBD there are associated behavioral difficulties. Many of these are because the child's problem has not been understood, causing him frequently to be placed under great pressure to perform in areas where he is unable to keep up with his peer group. This, of course, leads to the production of a very poor self-image and all its associated behavioral problems. Very frequently these children are hyperactive as well. They seem to be always in motion and their behavior is stimulus-bound (completely dictated by immediate surrounding stimuli). Although this tendency is greatly exaggerated by stress, many of these children seem to be overactive from birth. Some degree of motor awkwardness is also frequently present, manifesting itself in difficulties in handwriting, throwing and catching a ball, hopping, etc., all of which further complicate the child's life and serve as areas for potential stress. In summary, MBD children have difficulties in three main areas—learning, behavioral, and motor.

I have heard that there are special classes for children with learning disabilities. Can you tell me something about them?

Recently various school systems across the country have begun to develop special educational programs for children who are diagnosed as having organic learning disabilities or so-called MBD children. These are often referred to as special learning disability (SLD) classes, to throw in some more alphabet soup. Essentially these classes offer the child a much smaller pupil-to-teacher ratio and are far more highly structured than most "regular" classroom settings. Teachers who have been trained in teaching children with learning problems are assigned to these classes. Most of these children will later graduate or be phased back into the regular class situation, but in the meantime this type of placement can be of great value for many.

Are emotional problems commonly found in children with learning problems?

Yes, they certainly are. Any child with a significant learning problem is going to have some degree of emotional difficulty. Seldom does the emotional problem seem to be primary, however; behavioral maladjustment is usually secondary to an underlying organic learning difficulty.

Is it true that many adolescents with behavior problems may have learning disabilities?

Yes, we are recognizing with increased frequency that many of these persons have an organic learning disability that has previously gone unrecognized and underlies their emotional disturbance. The poor self-image, chronic frustration, and feeling of repeated failure stemming from an inability to progress normally in school is bound gradually to produce emotional disturbance, and although these behavioral symptoms may be the ones that draw attention to the child's plight, the underlying learning problem is likely to be the primary factor in their development. Many of the antisocial acts committed by teenagers and young adults, so-called misfits, have a learning disability at their base. Increasing attention is being paid to screening children with this in mind, rather than assuming that their problem is purely an "emotional" one.

HYPERACTIVITY

What is a hyperactive child?

This term, which has become very popular, essentially applies to the child who can't sit still. We all know at least one adult as well who fits into the same category. There is absolutely no objective or quantitative way to make this diagnosis. Hyperactivity is a symptom that is subjective and exists strictly in the eye of the beholder. The child who is described as being hyperactive by one person may not be so to another. Essentially he is a child who has a short attention span and is unable to focus on any one thing for more than a few seconds. He is constantly in motion and to be with him for even a short period of time leaves one exhausted! This type of child seems to lack the ability to shut out extraneous stimuli and his behavior is stimulus-bound. The truly hyperactive child is usually aware of his difficulty, and his inability to concentrate even when he tries his hardest is a source of great frustration to him, as well as to others.

Are all children with MBD hyperactive?

No, they're not. Hyperactivity has been in the headlines so much recently that one might assume that all children with learning problems have this behavioral characteristic. Nothing could be further from the truth, for many children with minimal brain dysfunction syndrome are underactive and many hyperactive children have no learning problems whatsoever.

My child has been diagnosed as hyperactive by the school and his pediatrician, who has suggested that we put him on medication. What do you think?

If your child has been carefully diagnosed as being hyperactive by several professional observers, he deserves some treatment, providing that his hyperactivity is significantly interfering with his school and/or social development. One should justifiably be skeptical when it comes to placing any child on medication, especially on a long-term basis, but in certain children drug therapy is indicated and may make the difference between success and total failure, not only academically but socially as well. To deny such a child a trial of medication seems to me unfair, especially since the potential benefits far outweigh the known risks.

What drugs are used for hyperactivity and what about their side effects?

Ritalin is by far the most widely used and efficacious drug in the treatment of hyperactivity. Fortunately it is relatively free of side effects. Your doctor will go over them with you before he begins any medication. Other drugs include Dexedrine, Benadryl, and several others. I have occasionally used Dexedrine but only if the child failed to respond to Ritalin since it has more side effects. No long-term adverse effects of Ritalin are presently known, but they could be found at any time. After all, we have used many medications for years before harmful side effects were brought to light, and one should always be cautious in using any form of medication.

What about dietary treatment of hyperactivity?

Recently, this has received a great deal of attention. In some children the removal of so-called food additives from the diet, especially those containing the salicylate radical such as artificial coloring, does seem to reduce hyperactivity. Unfortunately, keeping a child on this diet for a prolonged period of time is quite difficult and sometimes just about impossible. Chances are he will be unable to eat the usual school lunch, have a snack at his friend's house, eat at the birthday party, etc. Nevertheless, a trial of dietary therapy is certainly worthwhile, especially if it works! In my experience a small percentage of children who are hyperactive will be helped, but for the majority it isn't the answer.

OTHER LEARNING DIFFICULTIES

Is hearing loss sometimes a cause for learning problems?
Yes, it can be. Even a relatively mild hearing loss can produce difficulty in the classroom and result in personality problems. Every child with a learning problem should be carefully screened for any evidence of hearing loss.

The teacher mentioned that my five-year-old has difficulty with small-muscle coordination. What does this mean?
The term *small-muscle coordination* refers to hand movements such as those required in writing, cutting with scissors, tying shoes, and the like. The term *visuo-motor incoordination* is generally used to describe difficulty in coordination of eye and muscle movement and includes hand, foot, and general body motions.

What can be done to correct visuo-motor incoordination?
First of all, I think that this difficulty is vastly overdiagnosed, and many children who are just naturally a bit awkward receive this ominous-sounding label. Usually, with the passage of time, many children learn themselves to compensate or otherwise overcome their awkwardness. Currently much energy is devoted to various exercise programs designed to improve the child's coordination, but I know of no well-controlled studies that show such exercises improve the child's visuo-motor capabilities any more than would have occurred spontaneously as he matured. In addition, one must guard against labeling, and very often mislabeling, a child. Singling him out for some type of special program often does a great deal of damage to his self-image.

What is mixed dominance and is it a cause of learning problems?

Dominance refers to that part of the brain, left or right hemisphere, that is the dominant side for a particular function. For example, the speech center is most often in the left cerebral hemisphere. Cerebral dominance for hand function is also most frequently on the left side and the individual is therefore right-handed since the fibers from the brain cross over to the opposite side as they descend in the spinal cord. Most people are also right-eyed and right-footed. The fact that a child may be left-handed, right-footed, and left-eyed with respect to dominance does not mean that this is the cause of his learning problem or in any way contributes to it. It is true, however, that the incidence of learning difficulties in children with mixed dominance is higher than in those without, but no causal relationship has been found.

17

The Pediatrician and You

GENERAL

Should I take my child to a pediatrician?
Yes, I firmly believe you should. There is no other specialist
who is so thoroughly trained in the various aspects of child health
and no stronger advocate of his welfare. This is why most parents
continue to want a pediatrician to care for their child.

What is a pediatrician?
He is a physician who specializes in treating children, and
is responsible for their care from birth through adolescence. The
upper age limits vary with the individual doctor, but are generally
around 16. In addition to medical school, the pediatrician receives
a minimum of three years postgraduate training (internship,
residency). He may then take further subspecialty training in
some specific area of pediatrics, such as diseases of the newborn
(neonatology), disorders of the kidneys (nephrology), allergy,
neurology, and numerous others.

What does it mean when he is a board-certified specialist?
All physicians must take some sort of certification examination in order to qualify to practice medicine and obtain a license.
In addition, various specialty boards certify that the previously
licensed doctor has special competence in the specialty area in
which he is examined. The American Board of Pediatrics requires
the candidate to be the graduate of an approved medical school

and an approved pediatric training program. He must then pass both a written and oral examination before receiving board certification as a pediatrician. Because a physician is certified by the board it does not mean that he is any better a doctor than a pediatrician who is not so certified but has completed all the required training. The board certification does mean, however, than he has had to pass an extensive examination in the field of pediatrics and has been judged competent to practice the specialty.

Recently the American Academy of Pediatrics has instituted a program of recertification, which means that its members will be required to take periodic examinations throughout their professional careers.

How many pediatricians are members of the American Academy of Pediatrics and how may of these are in practice?

There are approximately 16,000 members of the Academy, of whom 12,000 are engaged in the practice of pediatrics. This is remarkable when one considers that the Academy was only founded in 1930.

I take my child to a group of pediatricians. Their office is always very busy. How do they keep everyone straight?

If they are like most groups I know, each doctor follows his own patients. When parents entrust their children's health care to you, it does not take long before you can remember individual children without difficulty. At times, when one doctor is on call, the others will fill him in with details about any child about whom they are concerned so there is no lapse in the continuity of care provided.

I take my child to a group of pediatricians. One is an allergist and the other specializes in neurological problems. Are subspecialties common among pediatricians?

Yes, they certainly are, and interest in the subspecialty areas continues to grow. The vast majority, however, practice general pediatrics. Only a small number (approximately 5 percent) limit their practice to the subspecialty area.

What are some of the subspecialties?
Allergy and immunology—Has its own subspecialty board for certification.
Neurology—Likewise a separate board for certification.
Hematology—Diseases of the blood.
Neonatology—Problems of the newborn; has its own subspecialty board certification.
Endocrinology—Glandular problems such as diseases of the thyroid gland, diabetes.
Nephrology—Diseases of the kidney and urinary system.
Radiology—Various X-ray procedures, both diagnostic and therapeutic.
Cardiology—Diseases of the heart and blood vessels; has its own subspecialty board certification.
There are others as well.

How many patients does the average pediatrician see in a day?
A recent survey conducted by the American Academy of Pediatrics found the number to be 29.

At what age does a pediatrician stop seeing children?
This varies according to the individual, but most of us like to carry our patients through the adolescent period. When you have known a child all his life it just makes good sense to follow him through those early teen-age years. I would say that the average age is around 16, but it varies a good deal. When the teen-ager begins to feel uncomfortable sitting in your reception room because of the presence of younger children, it's about time for him to move on.

COST OF PEDIATRIC CARE

How should I go about asking what the pediatrician will charge?
I am a firm believer in excellent communication between physician and patient at all times. This is the touchstone on which good medical care must be based. A good physician is well aware of this and should not take any offense whatsoever or feel that it is at all out of the ordinary to be asked about fees.

How do I know if what he charges is in line with the rest of the medical community?

One way is to check with some of your friends who have other doctors. Another is to check through your county medical society, which has a fee review committee and should be able to give you some helpful information.

Is pediatrics a highly paid specialty?

No, it ranks far down the list of medical specialties in this respect, yet it continues to draw plenty of graduate doctors into its ranks. Approximately 10 percent of each medical school graduating class enters the specialty.

DEALING WITH THE PEDIATRICIAN

We are moving to another part of the country. How should we go about finding another pediatrician?

Ask your present pediatrician whom he would recommend.

Ask your friends or people in the area in whom you have confidence.

Ask the local medical society or children's hospital.

Once you have settled on a pediatrician you will want to call his office to introduce yourself and make an appointment to bring your child in for a routine checkup. Don't wait until he gets sick. It's much better if your new doctor knows him beforehand, and if he has any special problems, such as drug allergies, heart disease, etc., it is even more important that he be familiar with him as well as with his medical record.

Are there any suggestions you would make about appointments for regular checkups for my children?

Call well in advance, as most pediatricians I know have a busy schedule; by planning ahead you can get the time you desire.

Be on time. I appreciate that waiting in a doctor's office is not a rarity, but if the office seems to run generally on schedule try to be there when you are scheduled to be.

Don't threaten your child with a visit to the doctor's office or with a "shot" if he acts up.

Familiarize him with what will be done before you come: "The doctor will look in your mouth," and you can demonstrate at home with the handle of a teaspoon on the tongue, etc.

Try to schedule infant examinations after feeding time so that the baby is not crying in hunger throughout the checkup.

How should I go about calling my pediatrician when I have a question or if my child is sick?

First of all, it is a good idea always to ask your doctor in advance how he handles his phone calls. Many pediatricians, myself included, have a call hour every morning. This time is set aside exclusively to answer questions, and, in addition, if your child is sick, it is a good time to check for advice or to make an appointment for him to be seen. During regular office hours the nurse or doctor's assistant may take your call and either provide information or put you through to the doctor if it is something that requires his immediate attention. Don't abuse this privilege since if he is not answering the phone, he is busy with a patient. You would not want your visit interrupted; neither does the parent he's with. If it is not an emergency, and the doctor's staff does not feel capable of handling your question, just leave a message. Trust the staff; they will give the doctor your message and he will check back with you. If it is a matter such as immunizations for foreign travel, behavior, or possibly a learning problem, he might not call until much later in the day, but be patient and trusting and he will appreciate your confidence.

What information should I have available when I call in?

If your child is sick it is a good idea to have a current appraisal of his status. For example, if you are phoning in the morning call hour and he got sick the night before, make sure that you have awakened him and judged the current status. If he feels warm or is sick, check his temperature and have the information available. It is also helpful to have pencil and paper ready to write down any instructions, as well as the number of your local drugstore in case the doctor wishes to prescribe some medication over the phone.

I am not fully satisfied with the answer my doctor gave me to the problem and still feel uneasy about it. What should I do?

You should discuss your doubts with him. Be honest and straightforward about it, and don't feel there is anything wrong with questioning his judgment. If you still feel in doubt, chances are he will either suggest a consultation with another physician or you may suggest that you would feel better if you had another opinion. There is simply no reason why you have to remain in doubt, and no harm is done in discussing your feelings with your physician.

My doctor seemed annoyed at me when I called him the other night and yet I thought the question was important.

I am sure it was an important question to you, but did you stop to think that you might have asked it during the call hour or the regular office day? Before calling your physician at night, just pause a moment and give some thought as to whether the call is really necessary.

Calls in the middle of the night that can be avoided:

The essence of any good pediatric practice is communication among parents, child, and doctor. This is in no way intended to inhibit that communication but instead to educate parents.

Earache—It is wise to have some sort of ear drops on hand. These plus aspirin and occasionally a hot water bottle or heating pad over the ear will almost always do until he can be checked in the morning. There are often a few drugstores open all night in case an emergency trip is necessary.

Pinworms—He may have some local itching, but don't panic. These are common and easily treated in the morning.

Prescription refills—Please remember to have it refilled during daylight hours when the pharmacy is open.

Fever—If the fever just started the same evening and there are no other signs of illness, this is not an emergency and it is perfectly reasonable to give aspirin, some sips of clear fluid, and check in the morning. (Infants under three months of age are an exception.) Every fever does not need to be immediately reported to the doctor.

Croup—Most cases are quite mild. If your child awakens with a barking cough, try using the vaporizer, and if this does not give relief then turning on the hot water in the bathroom and letting him breathe the moist air is usually enough to settle him down. Your being calm will help him. If he is able to get off to sleep, then his air exchange is adequate. If he continues to have trouble despite vaporizer and steaming, you will want to call your doctor no matter what the hour and he will expect you to do so.

Abdominal pain—Frequently children will have abdominal pain that will begin at night or it may awaken the child. If the pain is intermittent (comes and goes), it usually means the onset of some sort of gastroenteritis or intestinal virus. If it is constant and becomes progressively more severe, it may well be the start of an attack of appendicitis. It is perfectly safe to wait an hour or two to see if your child will settle down and go back to sleep. If something of an urgent nature is going on in his tummy, he won't settle down at all or will frequently awaken in obvious pain. This situation, of course, demands medical attention.

Head lice—They are pesky and can cause lots of itching but are not a medical emergency.

Cough, diarrhea, etc.—Almost always it is perfectly reasonable to treat your child symptomatically (with aspirin for fever and fluids for hydration) for the first few hours and often for the first 24 hours before checking in with your doctor. The onset of these symptoms during the evening or night is not an emergency situation.

Finally, "If in doubt, call," is a good rule to go by.

Suppose you are playing tennis. How can patients reach you?

Most physicians have an answering service during times when the office is closed. The operator knows where to reach your doctor since he tells her his whereabouts at all times. If he is temporarily out of reach of the phone he makes it a practice to check in with the operator on a regular basis, usually about every hour. Some physicians use a pocket-radio page system in which they can be alerted that the operator wants them to get in touch. In any case if you have an emergency don't wait—go directly to the nearest hospital.

My doctor is away for the weekend. What should I do?

He must provide coverage when he is away. Call the office number and inquire about what arrangements have been made. Usually you will be given the name and number of the doctor who is taking his calls.

Do you still make house calls?

Yes, but very infrequently. I really can't think of any situation where the child cannot be brought to the office or, if he is very ill, perhaps directly to the hospital. Nevertheless, I think that any physician should be willing to make a house call if he feels it would be the best way to handle the problem.

When I call my pediatrician, he so often says, "We have a lot of that going around." How does he know?

Since he sees many children and talks to many parents by phone, if there is an outbreak of an illness in the community he will soon know about it. He also meets and talks with other pediatricians in the community and compares notes. It is remarkable how similar the experiences will be. For example, if there is a sudden outbreak of gastroenteritis (the tummy virus), you can bet that all pediatricians in the area will be seeing lots of children with the same symptoms. As for the broader picture, several excellent publications help him to keep abreast of what is going on outside the immediate area. One of the best of these is a weekly publication of the U.S. Communicable Disease Center which gives the incidence in geographic areas of all types of infections throughout the United States.

My child had a checkup in March, his school just sent me a form for his September entrance, and he has another one for camp this summer. Will he need an additional checkup?

No, once a year is enough after age three. If you mail the forms in to the doctor's office they can be filled out with the data from his last examination.

My husband and I are planning to be out of the country and are leaving the children with a very capable sitter. Is there anything we should do to authorize treatment for the children while we are away?

You might want to check with your attorney on this matter, but I think it is helpful if you leave a notarized letter authorizing your pediatrician to provide medical care in your absence. You can rest assured that in an emergency situation he will, of course, be taken care of, but many times hospitals insist on proper authorization before doing minor procedures such as taking X-rays, putting in stitches, and the like and therefore some written authorization frequently will prevent a long and unnecessary wait in the hospital emergency room.

I have heard a lot recently about prescribing drugs by their generic names. Can you tell me something about this?

The generic name is the chemical name for a drug, as opposed to the brand name given the drug by the individual company that manufactures it. One antibiotic may therefore be produced my many different companies and will have many different brand names, but only one chemical or genetic one. Pharmacies can and do often charge less for drugs prescribed by the generic name because they can buy them wholesale at the cheapest price. Most physicians prescribe "generically" where possible in order to save the patient money, but in some instances, where a certain brand may be thought superior, he will prescribe it specifically.

What is the call hour?

This is an hour, from 8 to 9 A.M., which I set aside each morning for the purpose of talking with parents. It is a time when they know that I am available to answer the kinds of questions that are the basis for this book. No charge is made for this service and for the most part I thoroughly enjoy it, and I think our patients are grateful for it even though on a busy morning it may not be easy to get through. The popularity of the call hour has increased greatly over the past few years and it is now in use all over the country.

Index

246/ *Index*

Lead poisoning
  house paint and, 102
  pencils and, 96
Learning, *see* Education
Legs, of infants, 56, 57-58
  see also Orthopedics
Lethargy, 112
Lice, 131-32, 237
Liver function, 10, 11
Low-birth-weight baby, 9
Lumbar lordosis, 151

Masturbation, 105
MBD, *see* Minimal brain dysfunction
Measles, 94, 130, 135
Medic-Alert, 193
Medical problems/emergencies
  animal bites, rabies and, 132-33
  in childhood, 95-102; abdominal pain, 237; blinking, 91; blood in stool, 91; burns, 98-99; butterfly bandages, 101; cancer, 91; carsickness, 87; choking, 97; constipation, chronic, 91-92; emergency procedures, 101-2; epiglottitis, 101; facial cuts, 99; fever, head injuries and, 96; finger caught in car door, 99; foot odor, 88-89; immunizations and, 92-95; lead poisoning, pencils and, 96; scrapes and cuts, 95-96; soiling pants with stool, 91-92; stitches, cuts requiring, 100-1; swallowing foreign objects, 96-97; tongue laceration, 100
  in infancy: accessory nipple, 66; baby shot, reaction to, 45-46; bow legs, 56, 58; cephalohematoma, 61-62; circumcision, how to care for, 47; colds, 63; colic, 25, 32, 38; coughing, 63-64; crib death, 69; crying, normal and abnormal, 35, 36, 37, 112; danger signs in newborn children, 12; ears and hearing, 58-60 *passim;* enlarged breasts, 67; eyes and vision, 53-56 *passim;* exchange transfusions, 11; fever, 48; gums, lumps on, 65; hemorrhoids, 69; hernias, 67-68; hip dislocation, congenital,

57-58; inverted nipple, 67; jaundice, 10, 11, 12; nasal congestion, 63; protruding navel, 66; pyloric stenosis, 68-69; skin rashes, 48-51 *passim;* spinal sinus, 64; sunken chest, 64; tongue-tie, 64; umbilicus, how to care for, 47; vaginal bleeding, 65
  lead poisoning, house paint and, 102
  lice, 131-32
  medicine cabinet, what to store in, 102
  poison, 97-98
  ringworm, 131
  ticks, 130, 138
  toddlers, head injuries and, 85
  vomiting, how to induce, 97
  worms, 131
  see also Behavior; Illnesses
Medicines, given to newborn child, 6
Megavitamins, 111
Mental retardation, 5
Milk, *see* Allergies; Bottle-feeding; Breast-feeding
Minimal brain dysfunction (MBD), 225-26, 227-28
Mixed dominance, 230
Molds, allergies and, 187, 188-89
Molluscum contagiosum, 138
Mongolian spot, 65
Mononucleosis, infectious, 135
Mosquito bites, 195
Mother, early contact between child and, 7
Mumps, 94-95, 130

Nasopharynx, 167
Neonatology, 8-9, 233
Nervous system/disorders
  cerebral palsy, 198
  Down's syndrome, 199
  headaches and, 198
  head injuries and, 199-200
  of infants, tremulousness and, 60
  sleepwalking and, 199
  see also Convulsions; Education, learning disabilities
Nose
  bleed, 164-65
  discharge, 165